T0186073

Multiple Choice Questions in Pain Management

Rajesh Gupta

Multiple Choice Questions in Pain Management

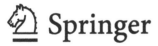 Springer

Rajesh Gupta, MD FRCA FFPMRCA EDRA
Consultant Anaesthesia and Pain management
Whipps Cross University Hospital
London, United Kingdom

ISBN 978-3-319-56915-4   ISBN 978-3-319-56917-8   (eBook)
DOI 10.1007/978-3-319-56917-8

Library of Congress Control Number: 2017948386

Printed on acid-free paper

This Springer imprint is published by Springer Nature
The registered company is Springer International Publishing AG
The registered company address is: Gewerbestrasse 11, 6330 Cham, Switzerland

Preface

A multiple-choice-questions book is not only meant to test the knowledge but also serve as a concise guide for revision. It should also be able to help save time acquiring the vast amount of knowledge from books. The purpose of writing *Multiple Choice Questions in Pain Management* is to provide the relevant information in an interesting format.

There are exit examinations all over the world after the pain fellowships for which there is no book available. This book also fills this gap for the trainees who are taking MCQ-based examination in the speciality.

This volume is divided into ten chapters. The chapters provide a systemic approach to chronic pain starting from anatomy and physiology to the complexities of specialised pain. The book starts with a chapter on basic considerations which is one of the most complex topics to understand. This is followed by the process of evaluation and pharmacological management especially the mechanisms involved. The book then discusses in detail the two main divisions of pain, somatic and neuropathic pain. The book further discusses specialised areas of pain like visceral pain, cancer pain and head and neck pain. The chapter on miscellaneous questions delves into specialised groups like pregnant population, paediatric population and elderly population. Effort has been made to frame questions based on evidence available in the literature. The highlighting feature of the book is detailed answers explaining the complex information in a format which is easy to grasp.

The book is not intended just to be a MCQ book but a concise pocket book explaining relevant concepts. It is meant for trainees but will serve an equal purpose for specialists who want to freshen their knowledge.

Rajesh Gupta
2017

Contents

Basic Considerations

© Springer International Publishing AG 2018
R. Gupta, *Multiple Choice Questions in Pain Management*,
DOI 10.1007/978-3-319-56917-8_1

❓ Questions

1. Coupling of action potential activity of C fibres:
   (a) Involves activation of one fibre by action potential activity in the another fibre.
   (b) Site of coupling is always near the receptor.
   (c) May contribute to flare response.
   (d) Is never seen in the peripheral nerves.
   (e) Frequently involves conventional C fibre mechano-heat-sensitive nociceptors.

2. Cold pain sensation:
   (a) Is mediated by both A and C fibres.
   (b) The sensation is subserved by deep structures.
   (c) Transient receptor potential ankyrin 1 (TRPA1) is the main receptor involved.
   (d) The threshold at which receptors are activated is 14 celsius.
   (e) The response increases with gentle cooling.

3. Chemical-induced pain:
   (a) Capsaicin induces pain on intradermal injection.
   (b) Capsaicin-induced pain is more when injected in the area of C fibre mechanosensitive receptors.
   (c) Capsaicin-induced pain is subserved by TRPV1 receptors.
   (d) Histamine causes itch sensation via C fibre mechanosensitive afferents.
   (e) Histamine-induced itch activates nociceptors via H1 receptors located in the peripheral terminals.

4. Hyperalgesia:
   (a) Threshold for pain is lowered.
   (b) Occurs only at the site of injury.
   (c) Heat hyperalgesia is coded by C mechanoreceptors.
   (d) C mechanoreceptors become sensitised in glabrous skin injury.
   (e) Pressure hyperalgesia is mediated by sensitised C fibres.

5. Hyperalgesia to mechanical stimuli:
   (a) Mechano-inhibitory afferents become hypersensitive after inflammation.
   (b) Response of only C mechanoreceptors is augmented with no effect on A mechanoreceptors.

(c) Receptor field is not affected.
(d) Spatial summation contributes to augmentation of pain.
(e) Injury to low threshold mechanoreceptors is one of the mechanisms.

6. Arachidonic acid metabolites:
   (a) Eicosanoids activate nociceptors directly.
   (b) Prostaglandins have no role in inflammatory pain and hyperalgesia.
   (c) Decrease in time interval between successive action potentials enhances the sensation of pain.
   (d) Leukotrienes also enhance the sensation of pain.
   (e) Cyclooxygenase 1 and cyclooxygenase 2 are induced in peripheral tissues by inflammation.

7. The following are true about inflammatory mediators:
   (a) Bradykinin does not have any role in nociceptive sensitisation.
   (b) Protons excite nociceptors without excitation or tachyphylaxis.
   (c) Histamine leads to a decrease in inflammatory peptides.
   (d) Capsaicin application reduces ATP-induced pain.
   (e) Increased levels of TNF alpha are seen in synovial fluid in the painful joints.

8. Nerve growth factor:
   (a) Is derived from mast cells and causes action by acting on mast cells.
   (b) Causes heat hyperalgesia by indirect action.
   (c) Alters distribution of mechanosensitive C fibres.
   (d) NGF-induced hyperalgesia is affected by TRPV1 and Na1.8 receptors.
   (e) Causes changes in nociceptor response properties.

9. Vanilloid receptors:
   (a) Are activated by capsaicin only.
   (b) Stimulation causes increase sensitivity in dorsal root ganglion neurons and primary afferent fibres.
   (c) Play critical role in cold hyperalgesia.
   (d) Protein kinase plays a significant role in heat hyperalgesia.
   (e) Inflammatory mediators can activate TRPV1 only directly.

10. Endothelin receptors:
    (a) Are present only in somatic tissues.
    (b) Endothelin 1 is released by endothelial cells only.

    (c) Peripheral stimulation of ETA receptors may result in hyperalgesia.
    (d) Activation of ETA receptors leads to enhanced excitability of
         nociceptors.
    (e) Endothelin has been implicated in sickle cell crisis.

11. γ-Aminobutyric acid receptors:
    (a) Activate both ionotropic and metabotropic receptors.
    (b) GABAa receptors are found in DRG cells.
    (c) GABAb receptors are found in primary afferents.
    (d) Activation of GABAb receptors by baclofen increases neuronal
         excitability.

12. Secondary hyperalgesia:
    (a) Present to both heat and mechanical stimuli.
    (b) Flare response contributes majorly to the phenomenon.
    (c) Does not spread beyond the midline.
    (d) Touch receptors may acquire the capacity to evoke pain.

13. Macrophages:
    (a) Play an important role in inflammatory and neuropathic pain.
    (b) Pentoxifylline reduces inflammatory pain.
    (c) Help regenerate nerve after injury.
    (d) Chemokine ligand-3 (CCL-3) blockade prevents thermal and
         mechanical sensitivity.
    (e) IL-10 reduces inflammatory cytokines.

14. Dendritic cells:
    (a) Are antigen-presenting cells.
    (b) Are called as Langerhans cells in the epidermis.
    (c) Play an important role in chemotherapy-induced peripheral
         neuropathic pain.
    (d) A number of Langerhans cells are decreased in skin of diabetic
         patients.
    (e) Are closely related to macrophages.

15. Cytokines:
    (a) TNF-alpha and IL-1beta can trigger inflammatory pain.
    (b) Antibodies against TNF-alpha and IL-beta are helpful in arthritic
         conditions.

    (c) TNF-alpha does not increase thermal hypersensitivity.
    (d) Leukaemia inhibitory factor (LIF) does not contribute to nerve injury.
    (e) IL-6 has a role as peripheral pain mediator.

16. Chemokines:
    (a) Are large molecules and are involved in immune cell recruitment.
    (b) CCL2 is upregulated in peripheral tissues in neuropathic pain.
    (c) Only act peripherally.
    (d) May release sympathetic amines from resident cells and contribute indirectly to hypersensitivity.
    (e) Get downregulated in peripheral nerve injury.

17. Nerve growth factor:
    (a) Acts on one receptor only.
    (b) trKA receptors are only present in periphery.
    (c) Animals born with lack of NGF are profoundly hypoalgesic.
    (d) NGF produces sensitisation of nociceptors by direct mechanisms only.
    (e) Elevated NGF levels are seen in inflammatory states.

18. Microglia:
    (a) Are derivative of macrophage population and invade and populate CNS.
    (b) P2X4-expressing microglial phenotype plays a key role in neuropathic pain.
    (c) P2X4R expression is only increased by CCL21.
    (d) Interfering RNA can block the effect of microglia.
    (e) Acute spinal application of ATP-stimulated microglia can cause hyperalgesia, allodynia and spontaneous pain.

19. Peripheral nerves that transmit pain:
    (a) Are characteristically small unmyelinated axonal fibres.
    (b) Primary afferent C fibres are lesser in number than myelinated primary afferent fibres in peripheral nerves.
    (c) The primary afferent fibres become the dorsal root.
    (d) Noxious mechanical, temperature and chemical information are relayed to ventro-postero-lateral nucleus.
    (e) The primary neurotransmitter substance in primary afferent nociceptors is substance P.

20. In spinal cord termination:
    (a) Sensory information is relayed uncrossed in the dorsal column.
    (b) Temperature and nociceptive impulses pass through the Lissauer's tract.
    (c) Small diameter primary afferents can be classified into peptidergic and nonpeptidergic.
    (d) CGRP is produced both by primary and secondary afferents.
    (e) Visceral afferents are rich in vasoactive intestinal peptide, bombesin, CGRP and substance P.

21. Spinal cord dorsal horn:
    (a) Contains both local interneurons and projection neurons that provide the information to higher centres in brain.
    (b) Both noxious and non-noxious stimuli relay across at least one synapse before reaching higher brain centres.
    (c) White matter is only composed of ascending fibre bundles.
    (d) Oligodendrocytes are the only glial cells unique to the CNS.
    (e) Projection neurons from spinal trigeminal nucleus terminate into ventrolateral nucleus of the thalamus.

22. Lamina of Rexed:
    (a) Laminae I and II forms superficial dorsal horn.
    (b) Laminae II to V are involved with tactile allodynia.
    (c) Lamina I contains 95% of projection neurons.
    (d) Substantia gelatinosa of Rolando comprises of laminae II–IV.
    (e) All neurons in lamina II are interneurons.

23. Lamina in the spinal cord:
    (a) Grey matter is a matrix of synaptic terminations and subdivided into ten laminae.
    (b) Somatic and visceral C fibre afferents terminate in laminae I and II.
    (c) Spinothalamic tract is formed of lamina I, IV and V projection neurons.
    (d) Scalloped primary afferent endings are seen in lamina II.
    (e) Visceral, nociceptive and autonomic processing area is seen in laminae III, IV, V, VII and VIII.

24. Spinal interneurons:
    (a) GABA interneurons are islet cells.
    (b) Glycine is the only inhibitory amino acid seen.

(c) Lamina II responds initially to substance P.

(d) Presynaptic inhibition is mediated by GABA interneurons.

(e) GABA B receptors can change their role from inhibition to excitation.

25. Projection neurons:
    (a) Three types of cells have been described.
    (b) Wide dynamic range cells respond only to mechanical stimuli.
    (c) Sustained nociceptive stimulation is required in all laminae to activate C-fos.
    (d) STT cells are affected by both excitatory and inhibitory events.
    (e) STT and interneuronal cells in the dorsal horn both express C-fos.

26. Projection neurons:
    (a) Mostly concentrated in Lamina I and scattered throughout III–VI.
    (b) Only have supraspinal targets.
    (c) Only the lamina 1 projection neurons are densely innervated by substance P containing primary afferents.
    (d) Hyperalgesia is mediated by NK1 receptor.
    (e) Waldeyer cells receive little direct synaptic input from primary afferents.

27. Spinal interneurons:
    (a) GABAnergic axons can be identified with antibodies against glutamic acid decarboxylase.
    (b) GABAnergic and glycinergic neurons are much more common in deeper laminae (III–VI)
    (c) Most GABAnergic and glycinergic axons form axodendritic synapses and generate postsynaptic inhibition.
    (d) Interneurons in lamina II are classified into islet cells, central cells, radial cells and vertical cells.
    (e) All the subsets of lamina II interneurons are GABAnergic.

28. Altered channel expression:
    (a) Nav1.8 activity reduction reverses nerve injury evoked pain states.
    (b) Systemic lidocaine can attenuate the hyperpathic state.
    (c) Mutations in Nav1.7 channel have no effect on pain sensation.
    (d) Loss of function mutations can cause erythromelalgia.
    (e) Potassium channel blockers increase ectopic firing after peripheral nerve injury.

29. Changes seen in injured axon:
    (a) Acutely TNF decreases potassium conductance in neurons while having no effect on long term.
    (b) Both application of TNF to nerve and systemic delivery result in hyperalgesia.
    (c) After nerve injury, stimulation of postganglionic axons will excite the injured axon and dorsal root ganglion of the injured axon.
    (d) Prostanoids increase the opening of TTX-insensitive sodium channels.
    (e) TTX-insensitive channels are typically found on myelinated axons.

30. Dorsal horn excitability:
    (a) Persistent large (A fibres) afferent activation has been shown to increase the receptive field of the activated neuron.
    (b) Persistent C fibre stimulation enhances the response to subsequent dorsal horn input.
    (c) As a result of persistent stimulation, enhanced response to subsequent dorsal horn input is seen.
    (d) High threshold tactile stimulation evokes a prominent response as a result of persistent C fibre activation.
    (e) Ongoing small afferent input can initiate central sensitisation of pain processing.

31. Free nerve ending receptors:
    (a) VR1 channel is responsible for inflow of sodium ions.
    (b) Injury/inflammation results in local release of inflammatory soup containing peptides, neurotransmitters (serotonin) and neurotrophins.
    (c) Substance P and CGRP are suppressed during the inflammation.
    (d) Local vasodilation and plasma extravasation are seen.
    (e) Activation of mast cells and neutrophils is seen.

32. Neuropathic pain:
    (a) Postherpetic neuralgia and chronic pain both are dominated by tactile allodynia.
    (b) Neuropathic pain may involve nociceptive input transmitted through nociceptive A-beta fibres.
    (c) Neuromas may generate spontaneous activity contributing to spontaneous pain.
    (d) Both A and C fibres show activity in nerve injury.
    (e) Neuropathic pain can develop in the absence of activity of injured nerve.

33. Central sensitisation:
    (a) Nerve injury induces upregulation of substance P and CGRP in layers 1 and 2 of spinal cord.
    (b) In cancer pain, galanin and neuropeptide Y are decreased.
    (c) Heterosynaptic mechanisms lead to allodynia.
    (d) Opioid receptors are upregulated in neuropathic pain.
    (e) Peripheral IL-1 participates in neuropathic pain.

34. Hyperalgesia:
    (a) Increased intensity of pain secondary to non-noxious stimuli is seen.
    (b) Can occur at a place distal to the site of the injury.
    (c) Isolectin B4 and VGLUT 3 are essential for induction of hyperalgesia.
    (d) Selective destruction of dorsal horn neurons that express neurokinin 1 leads to intense hyperalgesia.
    (e) Full expression of hyperalgesia requires intact lateral quadrant, lateral funiculus and dorsal columns.

35. Drug-induced hyperalgesia:
    (a) Abrupt withdrawal of opioids may contribute to it.
    (b) Opioid-induced hyperalgesia is presynaptic.
    (c) Consolidation and maintenance of opioid induced long-term potentiation involve presynaptic mechanisms.
    (d) Supraspinal sites have no role in opioid-induced hyperalgesia.
    (e) Drug-induced hyperalgesia is only seen with opioids.

36. Plasticity of inhibitory nociceptive pathways lead to:
    (a) Spontaneous discharge leading to paraesthesias.
    (b) Reduced inhibition of principal pain nerves leads to hyperalgesia.
    (c) Excitation in contralateral dorsal horn leads to radiating pain.
    (d) Spread of excitation from low threshold A-beta fibres to nociceptive-specific neurons leading to allodynia.
    (e) Rise in postsynaptic calcium levels.

37. Wind-up phenomenon:
    (a) Seen in response to temporal summation of excitatory postsynaptic potentials.
    (b) Ongoing C fibre discharges increase in incremental rate of five impulses per second.
    (c) It is a pathological process.
    (d) Long-term potentiation can cause stronger wind-up phenomenon.
    (e) Long-lasting changes in wind-up properties can be used as markers of plasticity.

38. Astrocytes:
    (a) Are the most numerous cells in the CNS
    (b) Are the only cells in the microglia that do not have a secretory function
    (c) Are essential for glutaminergic synapses
    (d) Are resistant to calcium levels
    (e) Synthesise and release pro-inflammatory substances

39. Periaqueductal grey matter (PAG) and rostral ventromedial medulla (RVM):
    (a) Contributes to hyperalgesia states associated with inflammation, nerve injury, immune system activation and stress.
    (b) RVM is required for hyperalgesia associated with naloxone-precipitated withdrawal or prolonged opioid administration.
    (c) Emotional affect associated with pain is provided by spinomesencephalic afferent to PAG.
    (d) Reversible inactivation with lignocaine into the RVM abolishes the analgesia produced by stimulation of the PAG.
    (e) Afferents from PAG to RVM are mainly serotonergic.

40. Sensory neurons:
    (a) Mainly originate from neural crest.
    (b) Survival of neurons depends on signalling from neurotrophin receptors belonging to tyrosine kinase family.
    (c) Migration of sensory fibres up to distal end of body continues till 10 years of age.
    (d) Each dorsal root ganglion innervates characteristic skin dermatome.
    (e) The number of dorsal root ganglion neurons increases with age.

41. G protein-coupled receptors:
    (a) Bradykinin, serotonin, prostaglandins and chemokines act on it.
    (b) Gs inhibits adenylyl cyclase.
    (c) cAMP effects are only mediated by phosphorylase A.
    (d) Gq activation can stimulate phospholipase c and PLA2.
    (e) B4 subunit of cellular function may be activated by G proteins

42. Nitric oxide:
    (a) Is an important extracellular mediator.
    (b) Is formed from L-arginine following activation of enzyme nitric oxide synthase.

    (c) Only the neuronal NOS is functional.

    (d) All the forms are expressed only in spinal cord.

    (e) Works by stimulation of cGMP.

43. Nitric oxide:
    (a) Actions are mainly spinal.
    (b) All the three forms are expressed in later stages of inflammation.
    (c) NO/cGMP activates sensory neurons by indirect mechanisms.
    (d) NO can stimulate dorsal root ganglion neurons by activation of TRPA1 and TRPV1.
    (e) Antinociception mediated by NO is mediated by inactivation of ATP-sensitive potassium channels.

44. Adenosine triphosphate:
    (a) Is released from damaged cells, and levels are increased in damaged and inflamed tissues.
    (b) Both Aδ and C fibres are excited by ATP.
    (c) Capsaicin increases the pain evoked by ATP.
    (d) P2X3 receptors may transduce ATP-induced nociceptive activation.
    (e) ATP antagonists are effective in reversing inflammatory thermal and mechanical hyperalgesia after nerve injury.

45. P2Y receptors:
    (a) ATP can stimulate sensory neurons by activating G protein-coupled P2Y receptors.
    (b) P2Y receptor-mediated excitation involves sensitisation of TRPV1.
    (c) P2Y1 receptor activation increases sensitivity to the TRPV1 against capsaicin.
    (d) Bradykinin sensitisation is mediated by P2Y1/2 receptor activation.
    (e) P2Y2 activation causes ATP-induced potentiation of TTX-resistant sodium channel (Nav1.8).

46. Adenosine:
    (a) ATP generates pain by releasing ADP, AMP and adenosine.
    (b) Is released from a variety of cell types.
    (c) Has no effect on sensory nerves.
    (d) Has only pronociceptive peripheral effect.
    (e) Prostatic acid phosphatase has antinociceptive effect.

47. Mast cells:
    (a) Granules contain histamine and can release cytokines and chemo-kines.
    (b) Chemicals in the granules of mast cells are pro-algesic.
    (c) Thermal hyperalgesia mediated by nerve growth factor is by its action on mast cells.
    (d) Antihistaminic treatment contributes to significant analgesia.
    (e) Mast cells can produce nerve growth factor.

48. Primary afferent signalling:
    (a) Shows ongoing activity in absence of a stimulus.
    (b) Responds only to chemical stimuli.
    (c) The frequency of firing in these afferents increases with the intensity of the stimulus.
    (d) Myelinated afferent axon leads to local increase in sodium current that depolarises the axon.
    (e) Menthol activates TRPV1 receptor to produce burning sensation.

49. Stimulus as a result of nerve injury:
    (a) Causes an initial burst of afferent firing.
    (b) Has an electrical silence for an interval of hours to days.
    (c) Appears over days of spontaneous activity in both myelinated and unmyelinated fibres.
    (d) Onset of pain behaviour follows weeks to months after the onset of ectopic activity in the neuroma and DRG.
    (e) Dorsal rhizotomy permanently abolishes the pain behaviour.

50. Altered channel expression:
    (a) Those that are resistant to sodium channel blocker TTX are found in Aβ fibres.
    (b) Is seen only in Nav1.8 and Nav1.9.
    (c) Potassium channels are downregulated after the nerve injury.
    (d) Potassium channel blockers are downregulated after the nerve injury.
    (e) Potassium channels carry the primary current for axonal depolarisation.

51. Toll-like receptors:
    (a) Are components of innate immune system.
    (b) Are only expressed in cells involved with immune function.
    (c) Mediate signalling with the help of cytokines.

(d) TLR4 agonists increase intracellular calcium and lead to release of neurotransmitters.
(e) Tenascin C can block TLR.

52. Neuropathic pain:
    (a) Pain of central origin can be because of direct insult to nociceptive pathways.
    (b) Complete lesion of dorsal roots causes severe neuropathic pain.
    (c) Neuropathic pain due to injury to PNS is more well characterised than due to central cause.
    (d) Inflammatory pain is not associated with tactile allodynia, heat/cold hyperalgesia and spontaneous pain unlike neuropathic pain.
    (e) Can develop in the absence of activity from the injured nerve.

53. Central sensitisation:
    (a) Inflammatory pain involves the sensitisation of both primary and spinal cord neurons.
    (b) NK1 receptor is inhibitory in inflammatory pain.
    (c) Both long-term and short-term inflammatory pain lead to burst of substance P.
    (d) The greatest change observed in the spinal cord in metastatic bone cancer is the activation of astrocytes.
    (e) Homosynaptic mechanisms are responsible for allodynia.

54. Placebo effect:
    (a) Is also seen in depression and Parkinson's disease.
    (b) Can be blocked by naloxone.
    (c) High placebo responders have increased opioid release in ventral stimulation.
    (d) Periaqueductal grey matter is involved in placebo-induced analgesia.
    (e) Opioid descending modulation with prefrontal cortical control of placebo analgesia.

55. Supraspinal degeneration in chronic pain:
    (a) Early hyperperfusion of the thalamus is seen in CRPS.
    (b) In Alzheimer's disease, higher levels of N-acetyl aspartic acid (NAA) are seen in parietal lobe.
    (c) Chronic pain is accompanied by cerebral hypertrophy.
    (d) Amygdala activity is increased in chronic pain.
    (e) Increased levels of IL-1β are a marker for brain regions undergoing synaptic plasticity.

56. Classic conditioning in pain:
    (a) Is based on Pavlov's experiments with dog and bell.
    (b) Conditioning in pain patients may lead to avoidance of behaviour previously considered normal.
    (c) Cognitive processes may interact with pure conditioning.
    (d) Conditioning may directly increase nociceptive stimulation and subsequently the perception of pain.
    (e) Repeated engaging in behaviour will be followed by a reduction in anticipatory fear and anxiety.

57. Operant conditioning in pain:
    (a) Is based on the fact that rewarding behaviour causes the behaviour to increase.
    (b) Pain behaviour includes overt expression of pain and distress.
    (c) Behaviour will occur more frequently only if it is positively reinforced.
    (d) Activity and working are helpful in decreasing pain behaviour.
    (e) Punishment and neglect may decrease the probability of behaviour recurring less likely.

58. Spinothalamic projection:
    (a) Originates from laminae I, IV–V and VII–VIII.
    (b) Spinothalamic tract (STT) cells are most numerous in thoracic enlargement.
    (c) Large population of STT cells is widely distributed in C1–C2 segments.
    (d) Lamina I cells innervate all tissues of the body.
    (e) Lamina I cells are present in the most superficial layer of the dorsal horn.

59. Lamina I cells:
    (a) Receive input from Aδ fibres.
    (b) Nociceptive-specific subtype has large receptive fields and responds only to innocuous stimulation.
    (c) Polymodal nociceptive subtypes get input from C fibres.
    (d) Thermoreceptive-specific lamina I STT responds to warming the skin and is inhibited by cooling.
    (e) All the subtypes are fusiform neurons.

60. Lamina IV–V STT cells:
    (a) Are large neurons in the neck of the dorsal horn.
    (b) Receive input from monosynaptic Aδ and polysynaptic C fibres.
    (c) Respond mainly to non-noxious mechanical cutaneous stimuli.

(d) Those having C fibre input can respond to activation with a wind-up discharge.

(e) Have large exciting fields.

61. Lamina VII–VIII cells:
    (a) Have widely radiating dendrites.
    (b) Respond to both noxious and innocuous stimuli.
    (c) Generally receive input from large diameter skin receptors.
    (d) Respond to both proprioceptive and visceral input.
    (e) Only receive large fibre input.

62. Posterior part of the ventral medial nucleus (VMpo):
    (a) Has the most dense STT termination field.
    (b) Serves as a thalamocortical relay nucleus for lamina I STT cells.
    (c) Lamina I cells are immunoreactive.
    (d) Is well developed in humans and non-primates.
    (e) Projects to the dorsal margin of posterior insular cortex in the lateral sulcus.

63. Ventral posterior nuclei:
    (a) Are dense along the rostral border of VP.
    (b) Have terminations from laminae IV–V.
    (c) Terminations in VP form ultrastructural triads with gabanergic pre-synaptic dendrites.
    (d) STT neurons that terminate in VP can have a collateral terminal in the CL.
    (e) STT input to VP has a role in pain.

64. Thalamic nuclei:
    (a) Ventrolateral nuclei are associated with sensorimotor activity.
    (b) Central lateral nucleus receives input only from laminae V and VII.
    (c) Central lateral nucleus projects to basal ganglia only.
    (d) Connections of parafascicular nucleus to MC are sensory.
    (e) Projections from lamina I also go to medial dorsal nucleus and from the project to area 24c in the cortex at the fundus of the anterior cingulate gyrus.

65. Spinobulbar projections:
    (a) Originate from same cells as STT cells.
    (b) Have termination in parabrachial nucleus.
    (c) Lamina I cells project to only reticular formation.

(d) A1 projections to hypothalamus are responsible for the release of ACTH and ADH in response to trauma and noxious stimuli.

(e) Lamina 1 input to parabrachial nucleus provides a substrate for integration of nociceptive activity with visceral afferent activity.

66. Trigeminal brainstem complex:
    (a) Receives input from nasal mucosa only.
    (b) Subnucleus caudalis is continuation of cervical spinal dorsal horn.
    (c) Clinical lesion leads to Wallenberg's syndrome.
    (d) Rostral trigeminal subnuclei can also be activated by orofacial nociceptive input.
    (e) Lesion of subnucleus oralis can interfere with nociceptive behaviour.

67. Gender difference in pain:
    (a) Female prevalence is higher in cluster headaches, pancreatic disease and gout.
    (b) Migraine is more common in females.
    (c) Rheumatoid arthritis pain symptoms fluctuate with sex hormones in females.
    (d) Irritable bowel syndrome symptoms are more in males than females.
    (e) Coronary artery disease pain is more in females.

68. Gender differences in pain:
    (a) Hyperalgesia is more common in females after inflammation or nerve injury.
    (b) Males are more sensitive as compared to females to noxious stimuli of common viscera in absence of injury.
    (c) There is conclusive evidence for higher incidence of most noxious stimuli during the follicular phase of menstrual cycle.
    (d) Hormone replacement therapy is associated with increased temporomandibular joint pain.
    (e) Anxiety appears to be more strongly related to experimental and clinical pain and treatment-related pain relations in men.

69. Gender difference in pain:
    (a) Women show greater antinociception from opioids.
    (b) μ-Opioid binding measures were found to be higher for females than for men in sacral brain regions.
    (c) Higher oestradiol condition leads to decreased in pain rating in females.

(d) μ- and κ-opioid agonists produce greater antinociception/analgesia in males than females.

(e) Nonopioid stress-induced analgesia is dependent on the NMDA receptors in males but not in females.

70. Affective disorders associated with pain:
    (a) Painful physical symptoms are seen in depression in 25% of patients.
    (b) There is more likelihood of pain causing depression than the other way around.
    (c) Ischaemic pain is felt more severely in depressed patients.
    (d) Hyperalgesia to heat pain in depressed subjects appears to normalise with duloxetine treatment.
    (e) Opioid treatment of pain in depressed chronic pain patients improves their depression.

✅ Answers

1. T T F F T
   Coupling is eliminated by injection of local anaesthetic thus indicating that the site is near the receptor, but it is also seen in peripheral nerves associated with nerve injury where it occurs at the site of axotomy. It normally contributes to flare response and efferent functions of nociceptors.

2. T T F T T
   The cold pain sensation is mediated by mainly A fibres but C fibres may be involved. Local anaesthetic application of the underlying vein abolishes the cold pain sensitivity. TRPA1 is mainly involved with intense heat and capsaicin.

3. T F T T T
   The response is weak when capsaicin is injected into C fibre MSA receptive area but is vigorous to A fibre and C fibre mechanically insensitive afferents.

4. T F F F T
   Hyperalgesia leads to reduction in threshold for pain, and pain in response to suprathreshold stimuli is enhanced. It occurs at the site of injury (primary hyperalgesia) and the area surrounding it (secondary hyperalgesia). Mechanoreceptors encode for heat hyperalgesia. C mechanoreceptors become sensitised in hairy skin injury. Pressure hyperalgesia is mediated by C fibres, whereas stroking hyperalgesia is mediated by low threshold mechanoreceptors.

5. T F F T T

Mechano-inhibitory afferent receptors become hypersensitive to inflammatory mediators like bradykinin, histamine, serotonin and prostaglandin E1 after the injury. Responses of both A mechanoreceptors and C mechanoreceptors are augmented after the injury. Receptor fields of both A and C nociceptors increase after the injury. Hyperalgesia to mechanical stimuli is due to injury to low threshold mechanoreceptors which causes central disinhibition of nociceptor input causing more pain.

6. F F T T F

Eicosanoides (prostaglandins, thromboxanes, leukotrienes) do not activate nociceptors directly but increase the sensation of pain by increasing the frequency of action potential firing. Prostaglandins are synthesised by Cox 1 and Cox 2 enzymes. Only Cox 2 enzyme is induced in peripheral tissues by inflammation. PGI2, PGE1, PGE2 and PGD2 are involved in inflammatory pain and hyperalgesia. LTD4 and LTB4 are involved in hyperalgesia.

7. F T T T T

Bradykinin acts on B1 and B2 to cause sensitisation by activating phospholipase c, protein kinase c and TRPV1. Protons are sensed by acid-sensing ion channels, and they cause excitation without showing any tachyphylaxis or adaptation. Histamine normally potentiates the response of nociceptors to bradykinin and heat. A subset of receptors (H3) is a ligand- gated ion channel that causes decrease in pain and inflammation by modulating the influx of sodium, thereby decreasing the inflammatory peptides. ATP-induced pain is dependent on capsaicin-sensitive neurons both in dorsal root ganglion and periphery. Increased levels of TNF alpha are seen in arthritis, and antibodies to the same can help ameliorate symptoms.

8. T F F T T

The sources for NGF include fibroblasts, keratinocytes, Schwann cells and inflammatory cells (lymphocytes, macrophages, mast cells). It causes heat hyperalgesia by acting directly on peripheral nerve terminals of primary afferent fibres. It alters distribution of A-delta fibres. It modulates the activity of ligand and voltage-gated ion channels involved in nociception (TRPV1, P2X3, ASIC3 and Nav1.8).

9. F T F T F

The Vanilloid receptors are present on primary afferent fibres and activated by capsaicin, heat and protons. The receptors play a key role in inflammation-induced heat hyperalgesia. A coupling is required with protein kinase A for inflammatory hyperalgesia. These receptors can be stimulated directly or indirectly (bradykinin).

10. F F T T T

Endothelin receptors are present both in somatic and visceral tissues. Endothelin 1 is released by endothelial cells, leucocytes and macrophages. The hyperalgesia effect is attenuated by endothelin antagonists. Activation of endothelin receptors on neurons results in enhanced function of TRPV1 and TTX-resistant Na channels and an increase in intracellular calcium levels leading to activation of PKc causing increased excitability of nociceptors. Endothelin has been implicated in sickle cell crisis, inflammation and skin incision.

11. T T T F

Both ionotropic (GABAa and GABAc) and metabotropic (GABAb) receptors are activated. The receptors inhibit neuronal excitability by inhibition of N-type calcium currents and potentiation of voltage-dependent K currents.

12. F T T T

Unlike primary hyperalgesia, secondary hyperalgesia is present only with mechanical stimuli. Flare response leads to spreading activation of nociceptors where activation of one nociceptor leads to activation of others. Secondary hyperalgesia does not spread beyond midline, whereas the flare response may spread beyond midline. Touch receptors may acquire the capacity to evoke pain because of central sensitisation.

13. T T T T T

Pentofylline decreases inflammatory pain by inhibiting the production of inflammatory mediators. Traumatic injury to a peripheral nerve results in degeneration of axons separated from their cell bodies and breakdown of the associated myelin sheath. Macrophages help clean up myelin debris which is detrimental to nerve repair. Blockade of CCL-3 reduces macrophage chemotaxis in acute inflammatory states thus decreasing hypersensitivity.

14. T T T F T

Dendritic cells also have phagocytic capabilities and can release cytokines and chemokines. In chemotherapy-induced peripheral neuropathic pain, Langerhans cells express OX-6 which is a marker of activation associated with pro-inflammatory cytokine production. Langerhans sells are increased in the skin of diabetic patients.

15. T T F F T
Both TNF-alpha and IL-1beta can activate and sensitise peripheral nociceptive neurons and contribute to ongoing pain and hyperalgesia. TNF-
alpha inhibitors like infliximab have been shown to decrease incident
secondary osteoarthritis in hands. TNF-alpha can enhance the sensitivity
of TRPV1 to increase thermal sensitivity. LIF belongs to family of neuro-
poietic cytokines and levels increase after nerve injury. IL-6 elicits calcium
transients in around 33% of DRG neurons.

16. T T F T F
CCL2 is able to elicit both thermal and mechanical hyperalgesia following
nerve injury. They can also act on dorsal root ganglion. Amines like CXCL8
and CXCL1 are released. They are upregulated especially CCL-2 which
recruits macrophages.

17. F F T F T
Two different types of neurotropic factors are there – low affinity NGF
receptor and tyrosine kinase (A, B and C). Forty percent of DRG cells express
NGF receptor trKA. NGF produces sensitisation both directly by activation
of trKA on nociceptors and indirectly by release of other algogens from a
variety of peripheral cell types. Elevated NGF is seen in inflammatory states
like bladder cystitis, arthritis and fibromyalgia.

18. T T F T T
Increased concentration of P2X4R is seen in the ipsilateral spinal cord with
peripheral nerve injury. P2X4R expression is also increased by IFN-gamma,
fibronectin, Lyn kinase signalling pathway and mast cells. Knocking down
of BDNF expression in microglia with small interfering RNA can abolish
the effect of intrathecally administered ATP microglia and pain behaviour.

19. T F T T F
Peripheral nerves are mostly C fibres with a conduction velocity lower
than 2.5 m/sec and A-delta fibres with conduction velocities of 4–30 m/
sec. The ratio of C fibres to A fibres is 2.5:1 in the dorsal horn, and in joints
it is 2.3:1. Sensory fibres form the dorsal root and motor fibres form the
ventral root. VPL nucleus of thalamus is the primary sensory integrative
relay of the sensory system. The primary neurotransmitter substance in
primary afferent nociceptors is glutamate.

20. T T T F T

Large myelinated afferent nerve fibres carrying sensory information like tactile, pressure, vibratory sense enters the dorsal horn and ascend uncrossed as white mater. Smaller myelinated and unmyelinated axonal fibres enter Lissauer's tract and then innervate grey matter. Peptidergic containing CGRP, SP and nonpeptidergic expressing purinoreceptors for ATP (P2X3) and binding Isolectin B4, CGRP-containing fibres can extend up and down and cross midline.

21. T F F F F

Only noxious stimuli relay across at least one synapse before reaching higher brain centres. White matter is composed of both ascending and descending fibres. Glial cells of CNS include oligodendrocytes, astrocytes and microglia. Trigeminal nucleus terminates into ventromedial nucleus of the thalamus.

22. T T F F T

Superficial dorsal horn is the main target for nociceptive primary afferents, and lamina II is further divided into Iii and IIo. Lamina I contains 5% projection and 95% interneurons; projection cells are larger than interneurons (marginal cells of Waldeyer contain glycine receptor-associated protein – gephyrin). Substantia gelatinosa comprises of only lamina II. Lack of myelinated fibres gives it a translucent appearance. It is here where the first order neurons of spinothalamic tract synapse.

23. Grey matter of dorsal horn includes laminae I–VI; laminae VII–IX and X are involved in somatic and autonomic motor function, respectively. Somatic C fibre afferents are located fully in laminae I and II, whereas visceral C fibre afferents terminate widely in laminae I, II, V and X. Scalloped primary afferent endings are large glomerular synaptic complexes seen in lamina II that contact multiple dendrites of dorsal horn cells.

24. T F F T T

GABA interneurons are found in laminae I and III and stain for inhibitory amino acid glycine. Dynorphin and glycine both are the inhibitory amino acids. Response to substance P is dependent on the presence of neurokinin 1 which is absent in lamina II. In intense prolonged nociceptive stimulation, GABA interneurons can override the inhibition and cause sensitisation.

Prolonged membrane hyperpolarisation can lead to it resulting in diminished presynaptic inhibition generating an action potential that travels to the periphery. This amplifies nociceptive input resulting in peripheral and central sensitisation thus promoting chronic pain.

25. T F F T T

Projection neurons are of three types – fusiform, pyramidal and multipolar. Both fusiform and pyramidal cells are nociceptive, while multipolar cells are thermoreceptive. Wide dynamic range cells respond to mechanical, thermal and nociceptive stimuli. C-fos is a proto-oncogene which leads to expression of dynorphin protein which is implicated in the development of pain state. Brief nociceptive stimuli cause activation in laminae I, IV and V, whereas sustained stimuli is required in III, V, VII and X.

26. T F F F T

Projection neurons generate local axon collaterals, thus contributing to inflammation in the dorsal horn. Apart from lamina I, lamina III–IV projection neurons express NK1 receptor and are densely innervated. Hyperalgesia requires NK1 receptor-expressing cells and not the NK1 receptors. Glutaminergic transmission from substance P plays a central role in the development.

27. T F T T F

Two isoforms of glutamic acid decarboxylase are seen – GAD 65 and GAD 67 – and are present in GABAnergic axons in dorsal horn. Only glycinergic neurons are common in deeper lamina. Islet and central cells have elongated dendritic trees; radial cells have short radiating dendrites. Vertical cells have dendrites that pass ventrally. Islet cells are gabanergic while radial and vertical cells are glutaminergic.

28. T T F F T

Nav1.8 and Nav1.9 are resistant to sodium channel blocker TTX and are found primarily in small dorsal root ganglion cells. Systemic lignocaine blocks ectopic activity and can attenuate hyperpathic state. Mutations in Nav1.7 can cause extreme pain while loss of function mutations can cause insensitivity to pain. Gain of function mutations can cause erythromelalgia.

29. F F T T F

TNF causes long-term effects through a variety of kinases (mitogen-activated protein kinases. Local application of TNF to nerve results in hyperalgesia, whereas systemic application results in decrease in pain behaviour. Prostanoids are eicosanoids consisting of the prostaglandins (mediators of inflammatory and anaphylactic reactions), thromboxanes (mediators of vasoconstrictor) and the prostacyclins. TTX-insensitive channels are found on unmyelinated axons.

30. F T T F T

Persistent C fibre stimulation increases the receptive field of the activated neurons. Low threshold tactile stimulation (wind-up phenomenon) leads to spinal sensitisation causing hyperalgesia and secondary hyperpathia (increased sensitivity to stimulus applied outside the area of injury)

31. T T F T T

VR1 channel gets activated at 43 °C and is sensitive to capsaicin and acidity.

32. F T T T T

Postherpetic neuralgia is dominated by tactile allodynia, while chronic low back pain is dominated with spontaneous pain. Neuropathic pain involves A delta and C fibres. Axotomised nerves develop terminal end bulbs, turn back on themselves and forms a neuroma. After nerve injury, C fibres show prolonged ectopic activity.

33. F F T F T

Nerve injury downregulates substance P and CGRP while upregulates galanin and neuropeptide Y. In cancer pain galanin and neuropeptide Y are unchanged while astrocytes are increased. Heterosynaptic mechanisms underlie the spread of hyperexcitability to neurons with input from intact afferents. Nonopioid receptors are downregulated in neuropathic pain while upregulated in inflammatory pain. Knockout of the proinflammatory IL-1 receptor along with overexpression of the IL-1 receptor antagonist decreases hyperalgesia and results in spontaneous activity from dorsal root fibres.

34. T T T F T

Hyperalgesia occurs at the primary and secondary site of injury and also spreads to the periphery. VGLUT3 (vesicular glutamate transporter 3) transports glutamate into synaptic vesicles. Selective destruction of dorsal horn neurons prevents full of expression of hyperalgesia.

35. T F T F F
Opioids suppress release of neurotransmitters from nociceptive afferents and on abrupt withdrawal; synaptic strength may remain potentiated for prolonged periods. Opioid-induced hyperalgesia is postsynaptic and requires activation of postsynaptic G proteins and postsynaptic NMDA receptors. Descending facilitation from brainstem sites plays a role in opioid-induced analgesia. Drug-induced hyperalgesia is also seen with ATP, BDNF and cAMP.

36. T T T T T

37. T F F T T
C fibre discharges at the rate of 0.5–5 impulses/second and then remains constant or decrease again. Wind-up phenomenon is an aspect of the normal coding procedures of some dorsal horn neurons. Long-term potentiations can cause higher amplitudes and longer duration of EPSPs leading to stronger temporal summation causing stronger wind-up.

38. T F T F T
Astrocytes account for 50% of glial cells in the CNS. They are highly secretory cells, encapsulate thousands of synapses of different neurons and are in contact with blood vessels. They are essential for glutaminergic synapses as they remove most of the extracellular glutamate. They respond quickly to elevated calcium levels. They may communicate over a distance by the spread of excitation through local nonsynaptic contacts referred to as «gap junctions». Astrocytes release IL-1beta, IL-6, PgE2 and NO.

39. T T F T F
Injection of lignocaine into RVM abolishes the analgesia. This is also achieved by anatomical lesions and microinjection of excitatory amino acid receptor antagonists into RVM. Afferents from PAG are mainly Gabanergic.

40. T T F T F
Migration of sensory fibres up to the distal end of body is complete by birth. The number of dorsal root ganglion neurons does not change but requires continued neurotrophin support.

41. T F F T T
Gs stimulates adenylate cyclase to raise the level of cAMP and activate protein kinase A in the neuron. cAmp can activate exchange protein and guanine nucleotide exchange factor.

42. F T F F T
    Nitric oxide is mainly intracellular. Three forms of NO are functional – neuronal
    NOS (nNOS), inducible NOS (iNOS) and endothelial NOS (eNOS). nNOS and
    eNOS are present at the spinal cord and brainstem, whereas iNOS is function-
    ally calcium independent and expressed in macrophages, inflammatory cells
    and glia. NO stimulates guanylate cyclase to produce cGMP which activates
    protein kinases, ion channels and phosphodiesterases.

43. T F T T F
    nNOS is expressed in early phase of inflammation while nNOS and iNOS
    are expressed in later stages. Antinociception is mediated by activation of
    ATP-sensitive potassium channels and inhibition of voltage-gated sodium
    channels in DRG neurons, which leads to inhibition of neuronal firing
    causing antinociception.

44. T T F T T
    Capsaicin decreases the pain response by desensitising the TRPV1-expressing
    fibres.

45. T T T T T
    P2Y2 receptors activation potentiates the capsaicin-induced TRPV1 cur-
    rents. P2Y1/2 receptor activation can increase the excitability of dorsal
    root ganglion neurons by inhibiting Kv7 potassium channels leading to
    bradykinin sensitisation. P2y receptors are a family of purinergic G pro-
    tein-coupled receptors stimulated by nucleotides such as ATP, ADP, UTP,
    UDP and UDP glucose. * P2Y receptors have been cloned in humans.

46. T T F F T
    Adenosine is released by endothelial cells, mast cells, neutrophils and
    fibroblasts. It can activate sensory nerves as intravenous administration
    produces pain in humans. Intrathecal administration of adenosine has
    analgesic effects mediated by A1 receptor activation. Antinociception
    mediated by prostatic acid phosphatase is due to hydrolysis of extracel-
    lular AMP to adenosine which stimulates A1 receptors.

47. T T T F T

48. F F T T F
    Primary afferents have no activity in the absence of a stimulus. Primary
    afferents respond to physical and chemical stimuli. Myelinated afferent

axon has specialised terminals that are sensitive to mechanical distortion leading to increase in sodium current. Menthol activates TRPMB (transient potential cation channel member 8) receptor and inhibits the sensation of low temperature.

49. T T T F F
Onset of pain behaviour parallels the onset of ectopic activity in the neuroma or DRG. Dorsal rhizotomy transiently abolishes the pain behaviour.

50. F F T T F
The channels that are resistant are Nav1.8 and Na v 1.9, which are found in small DRGs (C fibres). Altered sodium channels are Na v 1.8, Na v 1.9, Na v 1.6 and Na v 1.7. Sodium channels carry the primary current for axonal depolarisation.

51. T F T T F
Toll-like receptors are also expressed in macrophages, neutrophils, spinal cord neurons, glial cells and DRGs. Tenascin C is released in neuraxial tissue after peripheral injury and inflammation. Tenascin C is a glycopeptide and is expressed in the extracellular matrix.

52. F F T F T
If central insult directly involves nociceptive pathway, only than it is of central origin. Partial lesion causes neuropathic pain, while complete lesion has little chance of creating lasting pain.

53. T F F T F
NK1 receptors are expressed and internalised in inflammatory pain. Short-term inflammatory pain is not associated with burst of substance P and involves NK1 internalisation, whereas long-term stimulation involves burst of substance P. Allodynia is caused by heterosynaptic mechanism which underlie the spread of hyperexcitability to neurons' input from intact afferents leading to allodynia.

54. T T T T T

55. T T F T T
Early hyperperfusion in the thalamus might be a consequence of central sensitisation or spinal disinhibition as a result of apoptosis of inter-neurons. These changes are due to early activation of spinothalamic

pathway in CRPS. NAA is found in neurons, oligodendrocytes and myelin and is synthesised in mitochondria. Cerebral atrophy is seen in chronic pain which is caused by irreversible loss of neurons or by changes in volume. Changes in neuronal activity can result in cytokine induction in the brain and in long-term potentiation of synaptic activity in the hippocampus.

56. T T T T T

The experiments are related to stimulus associated with conditioning (dog and bell). A patient who develops increase in pain after physiotherapy may become conditioned and may develop negative emotions to physiotherapist and treatment room. Anticipation developed as a result of conditioning motivates a conscious decision to avoid specific behaviour or stimuli. Anticipatory fear can also elicit physiologic reactivity which may aggravate pain. Repeated engagement (exposure) produces less pain leading to decreased fear and anxiety.

57. T T F F T

Operant conditioning has been applied in pain by Fordyce. The main focus is modifying the frequency of a given behaviour. If behaviour is observable, it can make behaviour recurring. Behaviour will also be reinforced by escaping noxious stimuli with the help of drugs and rest. Pain behaviour may not be positively reinforced and more rewarding pain behaviour may be maintained.

58. T F T T T

STT cells are mostly located (more than 50%) in lamina I and the rest in laminae IV–V and VII–VIII. Most STT cells are located in cervical and lumbosacral region. Lamina I cells innervate the skin, muscle, joint and viscera.

59. F F T T F

Lamina I cells receive input from Aδ and C fibres. Lamina I cells have three subtypes: nociceptive specific (NS), polymodal nociceptive (PN) and thermoreceptive specific (TS). NS cells receive input from Aδ fibres, have small receptive fields and respond to noxious mechanical/thermal stimuli. PN cells respond to noxious heat, pinch, and noxious cold stimuli. TS-specific cells are divided into cool and warm cells; cool cells are stimulated by cooling and inhibited by heating the skin, while warm cells do the opposite. NS cells are fusiform cells, PN cells are multipolar cells, while TS are pyramidal neurons.

60. T T F T F

The cells receive input from Aβ fibres. The neurons respond mainly to noxious stimuli such as pinch, heat and deep squeeze. They are called wide dynamic range neurons as some cells respond to low threshold stimuli as well other stimuli like brushing hair or graded pressure. Wind-up discharge means that the neurons rapidly increase to a sustained plateau level if the stimulation is delivered at a rate faster than 0.3 Hz. These neurons are both excitatory and inhibitory stimuli.

61. T T T T F

Cells in the most medial intermediate zone, near the central canal (lamina X), also receive small diameter visceral input.

62. T T T F T

VMpo lies immediately posterior and inferior to the VP nucleus. The projection is well organised with lumbar input being most posterior and cervical and trigeminal inputs anterior. Lamina I cells bind avidly to calbindin which belongs to the family of calcium-binding proteins. The nucleus is well developed only in humans. The projections are the sensory representation of the body as insula is limbic sensory cortex associated with autonomic activity.

63. T T F T F

The terminations in VP neurons also stain positive for calbindin. Lemniscal terminations form ultrastructural triads with gabanergic presynaptic dendrites. STT input to VP nucleus has a role in sensorimotor integration.

64. T F F F T

Projections originate from laminae V and VII and VL projects to the motor cortex. Central lateral nucleus also receives input from cerebellum, substantia nigra, tectum, globus pallidus and motor cortex. Centrolateral nucleus also projects to superficial and deep layers of the motor and posterior parietal cortex. Connections to mediocentro nucleus are motor with connections to basal ganglia, substantia nigra and motor cortex.

65. T T F T T

Spinobulbar projections originate from laminae I, V and VII just like STT. They also terminate in regions of catecholamine cell groups, periaqueductal grey matter and brainstem reticular formation. Ventrolateral medulla has catecholamine cell groups (A1, C1, A5).

66. F T T T T
The complex receives input also from the teeth pulp, cerebral vasculature and cornea. Clinical lesions of trigeminal afferent fibres and nucleus caudalis at the level of obex can reduce orofacial pain and temperature sensation.

67. F T T F T
Female preponderance is seen in cervicogenic headache, limb pain, visceral pain and fibromyalgia. Migraine is more common in females (3:1) and in older women as compared to younger men. The duration is longer in females along with the intensity. Higher levels of anxiety and depression are seen in females in rheumatoid arthritis. Irritable bowel symptoms are about 55% in females as compared to around 37% in men. Female are older than men when seen for coronary artery disease. It is associated with pain in neck, back and jaw. Depression is seen twice as high as compared to men.

68. T F F T T
Stimuli of visceral pain are more prolonged in females and above the noxious threshold. Conclusive evidence of higher incidence of most noxious stimuli is seen only in electrical stimulation pain and that too in luteal phase. Oestradiol increases the excitability of TMJ afferents, which further increases following TMJ inflammation. It also alters gene expression in the trigeminal ganglion following TMJ inflammation. Discontinuation of HRT is associated with increase in musculoskeletal pain. Women report higher levels of anxiety sensitivity, which refers to fear of anxiety related body sensations.

69. T T T T T
Women also show significant hypoalgesic response to placebo. Opioid binding measure decreases with age in females. Higher oestradiol condition also shows greater μ-opioid activation in the thalamus, nucleus accumbens and amygdala. Oestradiol engages components of endogenous opioid system. Males express more μ-opioid receptor proteins in the spinal cord and midbrain as compared to females.

70. F T F T T
Painful physical symptoms are seen in 50–66% of patients and are an indicator of major depressive disorder. Ischaemic pain is felt alike in depressed and controlled patients, while thermal pain and paraesthesia is more in depressed patients.

Evaluation and Assessment

❓ Questions

1. Visual analogue scale (VAS):
    (a) Consists of a 10 cm horizontal or vertical line with end points as "no pain" or "worst ever pain".
    (b) Has no major advantage over NRS (numerical rating scale) and VRS (verbal rating scale).
    (c) Was developed to measure pain in domains other than sensory levels.
    (d) Standard VAS has no limitations.
    (e) VRS lacks sensitivity to detect changes in pain when compared with VAS or NRS.

2. McGill Pain Questionnaire (MPQ):
    (a) Fulfils all criteria of a just measure.
    (b) Provides us with an insight into the qualities of the pain.
    (c) Test-retest reliability coefficient of MPQ is very low.
    (d) VAS is more reliable than MPQ in measuring pain at the lower end of pain continuum.
    (e) The most valuable feature of MPQ is its use in differential diagnosis of various pain syndromes.

3. McGill Pain Questionnaire:
    (a) PainReportIt is better than MPQ.
    (b) Short-term McGill Pain Questionnaire is a short form of SF-MPQ containing similar descriptors.
    (c) SF-MPQ is not sensitive to any changes brought about by various therapies.
    (d) Full form MPQ distinguishes different pains.
    (e) SF-MPQ-2 was designed to measure neuropathic pain.

4. Pain measurement in elderly population:
    (a) VAS has best correlation with elderly population.
    (b) McGill Pain Questionnaire has validity in elderly population.
    (c) There is an increase in thermal and pressure pain threshold and decrease in pain tolerance with age.
    (d) C fibre and Aδ function increase with age.
    (e) In older population, pain at multiple sites is common.

5. Pain in elderly population:
    (a) Conditions that are excruciatingly painful in young adults may only manifest as behavioural changes in the elderly.
    (b) Postsurgical pain is seen more in elderly population.

    (c) Male gender is a strong predictor of severity of cancer pain in older patients.

    (d) Female gender is a strong predictor for chronic noncancerous pain.

    (e) Older people show lower levels of catastrophising.

6. Pain in elderly population:
   (a) The elderly are more specific targets for cognitive behavioural interventions.
   (b) Effectiveness of coping strategies and ability to control pain does not differ between old and young age.
   (c) Suicidal risk may be more in elderly population than young population in chronic pain.
   (d) Affective distress may be an important predictor of disability in elderly as compared to younger population.
   (e) Proportion of older patients who report chronic non-cancer pain differ by cognitive status.

7. Pain in children:
   (a) VAS can be reliably used in children >3 years of age.
   (b) Oucher scale is designed to measure pain intensity in children aged 3–12 years.
   (c) Girls >8 are more likely to complete pain diaries than boys for similar age group.
   (d) Touching the affected area of painful stimulus can be seen as early as 2 years of age.
   (e) Boys cry more as compared to girls in response to heel lance prick.

8. Pain in children:
   (a) CHEOPS scale is sensitive to changes after the intravenous injection of opioids.
   (b) FLACC scale is recommended for post-operative pain in children.
   (c) COMFORT scale is usually used in critical care settings.
   (d) Post-operative pain measure for parents has been validated in children as young as 2 years.
   (e) Infant pain behaviour rating scale has satisfactory inter-rater variability for most of the items.

9. Pain beliefs:
   (a) Individuals with high self-efficacy report low levels of disability and depression.
   (b) Acceptance of pain leads to more disability.

    (c) Fear avoidance can lead to more disability in conditions like fibromyalgia and osteoarthritis.

    (d) Catastrophising may have beneficial effect on pain-related function and depressive symptoms in months immediately following an amputation.

    (e) Distraction and ignoring pain has conclusive role in chronic pain management.

10. Brain activity associated with hypnosis:
    (a) Most consistent activity is found in theta range (4–8 Hz).
    (b) Subjects with high hypnotic susceptibility display more theta activity.
    (c) Hypnotic states are associated with decreased neural activity in occipital and anterior cingulate areas.
    (d) Anterior insula and posterior parietal cortex are important for self-agency in hypnosis.
    (e) Highly hypnotisable subjects also display hypnosis-induced decrease in EEG coherence between the midline frontal and lateral areas in the gamma band.

11. Chronic opioid treatment:
    (a) Tolerance to all side effects is seen.
    (b) Analgesic tolerance does not develop in cancer-related pain.
    (c) Use of opioids in chronic non-cancer pain is associated with more side effects.
    (d) Oxycodone has more risk of addictive behaviour than morphine.
    (e) In opioid-dependant patients, pain can coexist with high levels of exogenous opioids.

12. Addiction:
    (a) Is seen more in hospitalised patients receiving chronic opiates.
    (b) Is mediated by dopaminergic neurons of the midbrain ventral tegmental area.
    (c) Striatonigral connections are important for early response to drug intake.
    (d) Depletion of dopamine decreases subject's motivation.
    (e) Euphoria and well-being following opiate administration is because of dopamine release.

13. Addiction to opioids:
    (a) Aversive state of withdrawal is strengthened by repeated drug taking.
    (b) Salience theory proposes that sensitisation leads to a prolonged change in dopaminergic function that results in a change in the "wanting" rather than "liking" the drug.
    (c) Drugs with addiction potential increase dopamine in mesolimbic system principally through AMPA glutamate receptors.
    (d) Long-term habit forming is mediated by CREB.
    (e) Morphine agonists work by inhibition of ventral tegmental area dopamine neurons.

14. Addiction:
    (a) Dopamine release is decreased with opioids in chronic or neuropathic pain.
    (b) Dysfunctional activity is seen in prefrontal cortex (PFC).
    (c) Chronic substance misuse leads to decrease in dopamine response.
    (d) Post-acute withdrawal period may be followed by anhedonia and depression.
    (e) Relapse is due to neuroplastic changes in brain.

15. Placebo effect:
    (a) Can be created through conditioning.
    (b) Is seen only in somatic pain.
    (c) Causes a decrease in endogenous opioid and dopamine systems.
    (d) Involves contralateral anterior insula, medial thalamus and ventral dorsal cingulated.
    (e) Conditioning can produce negative expectation and brain changes that increase pain.

✅ Answers
1. T F T F T
   Patients place a mark on 10 cm line corresponding to the intensity of the pain. It is a numeric index of the severity of pain. Major advantage of VAS is its ratio scale properties. Equality of ratios is applied which makes it more appropriate. VAS has limitations in patients having perceptual-motor problems, clinical settings not suitable, or problems with telephonic surveys. The main disadvantage of VAS, NRS and VRS is the assumption that pain is a one-dimensional experience that can be measured with a single item.

2. T T F F T

   Just criteria include valid, reliable, consistent and useful. Test-retest coefficient is high and has very strong association especially with chronic pain syndromes that remain stable over time. MPQ is more reliable because of the multidimensional nature and large number of descriptors to choose from.

3. F F F T F

   PainReportIt is a computer tablet version of MPQ. It lacks three main indices of MPQ – (a.) sensory, affective and evaluative; (b.) total number of words chosen and (c.) present pain integrity. The word "splitting" was added to 15 descriptors as it was deemed a key word in dental pain. SF-MPQ is sensitive to analgesic drugs, epidurally or spinally administered drugs, TENS, acupuncture and low power light therapy. SF-MPQ-2 was designed to measure both neuropathic and nonneuropathic pain. The modifications include seven new descriptors relevant to neuropathic pain, use of an 11-point NRS for each descriptor, addition of qualifier pain to 13 descriptors, measurement of different qualities of pain and relevant symptoms.

4. F T T F T

   VAS has poor convergent validity and lack of agreement with other intensity measures. The elderly may find it difficult to complete VAS. MPQ's psychotomimetic properties are not age related, and it is also sensitive for the assessment of age and time-related changes in post-operative pain. There is no change in sensitivity to electrical stimulation and increased sensitivity to ischaemic pain. Both the fibres show decreased activity with ageing and also prolonged hyperalgesia is seen.

5. T T F T T

   Excruciating pain may manifest as confusion, restlessness, aggression, anorexia and fatigue in the elderly. Indicators of severity in cancer patients are female gender, younger age, advanced disease, no analgesic use, lower social support and depressed mood. Older people show low levels of catastrophising along with a low fear of pain and pain avoidance.

6. T T T F F

   Fear of reinjury may play an important role in depression and disability in older than in younger patients thus making them potential targets for CBT. Affective distress is an important predictor of disability in younger population, and pain severity is an important predictor of disability in elderly as compared to younger population.

7. F T F F T
    VAS has validity for children more than 5 years. Vertical scale is more appro-
    priate than horizontal as the concept of more or less is easier to grasp with
    up and down direction. Oucher scale is a variant of face scale and is sensi-
    tive to analgesia-induced reduction in pain. Variants of scale are available
    for African American and Hispanic children. Boys are more likely to com-
    plete pain diaries. Boys cried sooner and had more crying cycles.

8. T T T T T
    CHEOPS scale measures six expressions – crying, facial expressions, ver-
    bal expression, torso position, touch position and leg position. FLACC
    scale: face, legs, activity, cry and consolability. COMFORT scale reports
    alertness, calmness, agitation, respiration, physical movement, change
    in blood pressure, changes in heart rate, muscle tone and facial tension.
    Post-operative pain measure for parents measures pain than anxiety.

9. T F T T F
    Patients with higher levels of self-efficacy benefit most from self-management
    interventions. Acceptance of pain leads to less avoidance and less disability.
    Fear avoidance is measured with Tampa Scale of Kinesiophobia. Distraction
    and ignoring pain has conclusive role in acute pain management.

10. T T F T T
    Hypnosis has been associated with alpha activity with left hemisphere
    beta activity or with 40 Hz activity. There is an increased activity in occipi-
    tal and anterior cingulate areas, and decreased activity is seen in ponto-
    mesencephalic brainstem, medial thalamus and rostral anterior cingulate
    gyrus. Self-agency is a feeling that oneself is the agent of self-generated
    actions or mental processes.

11. F T T F T
    Tolerance is seen to nausea, vomiting, sedation and respiratory depression
    but not to constipation. Opioids have been associated with poor quality of
    life and functional disturbances.

12. F T F T T
    Addiction is seen in only 0.01% of hospitalised patients. Addiction risk
    with short-term opioid treatment is 3/1000. Early response to drug intake
    is mediated by VTA-ventral striatum, whereas change from voluntary to
    habitual use is because of more dorsal regions of striatum mediated by
    striatonigral connections.

13. T T T T F

Addiction leads to changes in mesolimbic system terminating with the nucleus accumbens. cAMP response element binding (CREB) protein is a transcription factor which has a role in neuronal plasticity. Initial movements are restricted with release of CREB in hippocampus, but habit forming causes a shift to dorsal stria which plays an important part in habit forming. Morphine agonists activate ventral tegmental area dopamine neurons and increase release of dopamine in the nucleus accumbens via inhibition of GABA in VTA. Acute administration of opiates leads to inhibition of cAMP pathway, whereas chronic administration leads to increase in cAMP.

14. T T T T T

PFC dysfunction is thought to impair impulse control. It also leads to lack of awareness of addiction. Abstinence leads increase in levels of ACTH, corticosterone, noradrenaline, neuropeptide Y and corticotrophin release factor. Endogenous systems take months to normalise causing insomnia, anxiety, depression, inability to concentrate, clumsiness and distorting dreams.

15. T F F T T

Placebo effect is seen in dental post-operative pain, post-thoracotomy pain, low back pain, IBS pain and chronic neuropathic pain. Nocebo effect produces negative expectation and brain changes that increase pain. The effect may produce stronger physiological responses such as cortisol.

Pharmacology

© Springer International Publishing AG 2018
R. Gupta, *Multiple Choice Questions in Pain Management*,
DOI 10.1007/978-3-319-56917-8_3

Questions

1. Opioid receptors:
   (a) Belong to superfamily of G protein-coupled receptors (GPCR).
   (b) Extracellular loops are similar in mu, delta and kappa receptors.
   (c) Extracellular domains of opioid receptors are considered to be both anchoring points for opioid ligands and gates filtering opioid entry into the binding pocket.
   (d) Transmembrane domain forms similar opioid-binding pockets across mu, delta and kappa receptors.
   (e) Helix of transmembrane domain is water accessible.

2. Opioid receptor signalling:
   (a) Is coupled to Gi/Go inhibitory proteins.
   (b) Involves activating calcium channels.
   (c) Involves activation of mitogen-activated protein kinase cascades.
   (d) Involves stimulation of G protein-independent signalling pathways.
   (e) Will lead to recycling of mu receptors to the cell surface.

3. Opioid-induced analgesia:
   (a) Kappa receptor-mediated analgesia is independent from mu and delta receptor-mediated analgesia.
   (b) Both mu and delta receptors are recruited in spinal and supraspinal analgesia.
   (c) Ablation of delta receptors causes an increase in mechanical nociception and inflammatory pain.
   (d) Delta receptor knockout leads to insensitivity to nortriptyline.
   (e) Prodynorphin has a biphasic role in control of nociceptive responses.

4. Spinal analgesia with opioids:
   (a) Opioid receptors are located mostly in superficial dorsal horn.
   (b) Opioid binding to receptors is maximally seen with kappa receptors.
   (c) Spinally applied morphine can reduce release of substance P and calcitonin G.
   (d) Predominant site of spinal opioid action is via presynaptic opioid receptors on the central terminals of nociceptive afferents.
   (e) Opioids control dynamic allodynia better than noxious and static allodynia.

5. Supraspinal analgesia:
   (a) Main sites for opioid action are midbrain and brainstem structures.
   (b) Nitric oxide is important for 5HT-mediated inhibition of PAG output and reversal of antinociception.
   (c) Fibres descending from PAG to dorsal horn of spinal cord are mainly GABAnergic.
   (d) Opioids can also interfere with noradrenergic mechanisms.
   (e) Tramadol is a weak opioid.

6. Opioids in neuropathic pain:
   (a) Both static and dynamic allodynia are seen after nerve injury.
   (b) Static allodynia is dependent on capsaicin-dependent Aδ fibres.
   (c) Morphine blocks static allodynia when administered spinally in nerve injuries.
   (d) Large A fibres do not possess opioid receptor.
   (e) Nerve injury leads to increased transmitter release via calcium channels.

7. Codeine:
   (a) Is metabolised in liver.
   (b) In a dosage of 60 mg, it is a good analgesic by itself.
   (c) Is as potent as ibuprofen.
   (d) Has a NNT of 8.1.
   (e) In a dosage of 30 mg, it improves analgesic efficacy of nonopioids.

8. Tramadol:
   (a) Has an oral bioavailability of 80–90%.
   (b) Has dose-dependent analgesic efficacy.
   (c) Has good efficacy for neuropathic pain.
   (d) Has high potential for addiction.
   (e) Has a low risk of respiratory depression.

9. Morphine:
   (a) Has an oral bioavailability of 10–45%.
   (b) Has active metabolites that contribute to analgesia.
   (c) Should be avoided in renal impairment.
   (d) Low release formulation has better analgesic profile than immediate release formulation.
   (e) Has a NNT of 2.9 for intramuscular route.

10. Oxycodone:
    (a) Is a semisynthetic derivative of thebaine.
    (b) Has less bioavailability than morphine.
    (c) Has a better NNT for neuropathic pain than TCAs.
    (d) Is only effective for somatic pain.
    (e) Has less complications than morphine.

11. Methadone:
    (a) Is a synthetic opioid used in opioid addiction.
    (b) Is contraindicated in hepatic and renal impairment.
    (c) Steady-state plasma concentration may take 10 days to achieve.
    (d) Has a short half-life.
    (e) May prolong QTc interval.

12. Methadone:
    (a) Is a racemic mixture of two enantiomers.
    (b) Has a higher affinity for delta receptors than morphine.
    (c) Has a long half-life.
    (d) Has a reduced clearance in acidic urine.
    (e) Increases QTc interval.

13. Fentanyl:
    (a) Is a potent kappa agonist.
    (b) Is ideal for transmucosal and transdermal administration.
    (c) Has a poor systemic level after transdermal administration.
    (d) Is available only for intravenous administration.
    (e) Has high risk of abuse.

14. Route of administration of opioids:
    (a) Bioavailability of fentanyl is higher than morphine via sublingual route.
    (b) Intranasal preparations are mainly used for breakthrough pain.
    (c) Morphine by inhalation route has a bioavailability of 55%.
    (d) Fentanyl iontophoretic patches have technical difficulties in the form of corrosion.
    (e) Subcutaneous route is mainly used for cancer pain.

15. Short-term side effects of opioids:
    (a) Tolerance to respiratory depression does not occur.
    (b) Nausea and vomiting occurs due to direct effect on chemoreceptor trigger zone in area postrema of medulla.

   (c) Tolerance to sedation develops quickly.
   (d) Both visual and tactile hallucinations can be seen.
   (e) Clonazepam is the medication of choice for opioid-induced seizures.

16. Adverse effects of long-term use of opioids:
   (a) Tolerance develops only on long-term usage.
   (b) Physical dependence may be seen on acute administration.
   (c) Addiction is not seen with acute/cancer pain management.
   (d) Intramuscular route is ideal for post-operative pain relief.
   (e) Tramadol is a safe alternative in patients at risk for opioid side effects.

17. Opioids:
   (a) Receptors are located mainly in the dorsal horn of the spinal cord.
   (b) Receptors are located only on presynaptic sites.
   (c) Receptors mainly modulate visceral pain.
   (d) Undergo hepatic metabolism.
   (e) Are mainly metabolised by CYP-2D6 and its absence is seen in 50% of white population.

18. Opioids:
   (a) Morphine and methadone achieve steady-state concentration in 24 h.
   (b) Methadone is useful in short gut syndrome.
   (c) Tolerance to constipation does not develop.
   (d) Treatment of opioid-induced constipation is stool softeners and fibre-based bulking agents.
   (e) Alvimopan acts as a peripherally acting mu opioid antagonist.

19. Complications of opioids:
   (a) Pruritus is seen more via intravenous/neuraxial route.
   (b) Pruritus is because of histamine release.
   (c) Fentanyl does not have active metabolites so it causes less sedation.
   (d) Respiratory depression may be delayed for as much as 12 h after neuraxial administration.
   (e) Naloxone administration can cause congestive heart failure with seizures.

20. Opioids:
   (a) Cause reduction in immune function.
   (b) Cause sexual dysfunction only in men.
   (c) Has no effect on sleep architecture.
   (d) Tolerance involves NMDA receptors.
   (e) Tolerance can be treated by opioid rotation.

21. Opioid side effects:
    (a) Noradrenergic neurons within locus coeruleus are implicated in the maintenance of dependence.
    (b) Addiction is mediated by ventral tegmental dopaminergic area and orbitofrontal glutaminergic projections to nucleus accumbens.
    (c) Alpha2 agonists and beta-agonists can attenuate many of the symptoms of opioid withdrawal.
    (d) Withdrawal symptoms usually last for 1 month.
    (e) Clonidine can help in weaning from opioids.

22. Codeine:
    (a) Is similar in affinity for mu opioid receptors as is morphine.
    (b) Is converted to morphine by O-demethylation.
    (c) Major enzyme for conversion to morphine is CYP2D6.
    (d) NNT of codeine (60 mg) is 17.
    (e) Works more effectively in combination.

23. Acetaminophen:
    (a) Paracetamol (active metabolite of phenacetin) has fewer side effects.
    (b) Works by inhibiting prostaglandin formation.
    (c) Causes central analgesic effects due to decrease in beta-endorphins.
    (d) Is metabolised mostly by renal pathway.
    (e) Toxicity is increased with low glutathione levels.

24. Acetaminophen-induced toxicity:
    (a) Causes depletion of glutathione stores.
    (b) Is seen with dosages increasing 1 g.
    (c) Can be seen within daily normal dosages in the form of increased alanine transaminase levels.
    (d) Is increased by concomitant usage of alcohol.
    (e) Can cause hypertension.

25. Tramadol:
    (a) Has central analgesic properties.
    (b) Mainly involves mu receptors and effects are fully antagonised by naloxone.
    (c) Has equal bioavailabilities for both extended release and immediate release formulations.
    (d) Has maximum bioavailability via rectal route.
    (e) Has more side effects with extended release formulation.

26. Oral steroids:
    (a) Exert analgesic effects through strong anti-inflammatory actions.
    (b) Are readily absorbed through gastrointestinal tract.
    (c) Have bone fractures as main side effects.
    (d) May have a role in chemotherapy-induced peripheral neuropathy.
    (e) Are of benefit in disc interruptions.

27. Topical medications:
    (a) NNT for steroids is more for acute pain than chronic pain.
    (b) Topical ketoprofen has the best analgesic profile of all topical NSAIDs.
    (c) Lidocaine patches work by binding to and blocking the sodium channels.
    (d) TRPV1 receptors are only activated by capsaicin.
    (e) Menthol provides analgesia only by its calcium-blocking actions.

28. Topical analgesics:
    (a) Five percent lidocaine patch is as effective as pregabalin in postherpetic neuralgia.
    (b) Five percent lidocaine has no role in postherpetic neuralgia.
    (c) Eight percent capsaicin patch has efficacy in postherpetic neuralgia and painful HIV neuropathy.
    (d) Topical flurbiprofen has greater pain reduction than topical diclofenac.
    (e) Topical diclofenac has similar efficacy as oral diclofenac.

29. Cyclooxygenases:
    (a) Convert arachidonic acid into prostaglandin G2 and H2.
    (b) COX-1 is induced only in response to inflammatory stimuli.
    (c) COX-2 inhibition may increase the risk of hypertension and increase cardiovascular risk.
    (d) Aspiring/acetylsalicylic acid permanently inhibits COX inhibitors.
    (e) COX-3 is present in humans.

30. Cyclooxygenases:
    (a) Prostaglandins act on voltage-gated sodium channels.
    (b) Thermal hyperalgesia in inflammatory diseases is mediated by cyclooxygenases.
    (c) Prostaglandins increase the excitability of nociceptive nerve fibres.
    (d) Intrathecal ketorolac can reduce spinal PGE2 levels.
    (e) Inhibition of platelet aggregation is mediated by prostaglandins.

31. Cyclooxygenases:
    (a) Blockade of COX-2 reduces tissue concentration of prostanoids and also increases endocannabinoids.
    (b) Indomethacin has analgesic effect due to increase in spinal endocannabinoids.
    (c) Anti-inflammatory action of aspirin-triggered lipoxins is mediated by COX-2 inhibitors.
    (d) Non-acidic compounds have high lipophilicity and can enter the CNS.
    (e) Ibuprofen is used as an S enantiomer.

32. NSAIDs:
    (a) Diclofenac works equally well on COX-1 and COX-2.
    (b) Galenic formulation of the drug increases absorption of diclofenac.
    (c) Diclofenac has significant first-pass metabolism.
    (d) Liver toxicity is not seen with diclofenac.
    (e) Post-operative bleeding may be seen with ketorolac.

33. Aspirin:
    (a) Inactivates both COX enzymes permanently.
    (b) Has no effect on thrombocytes.
    (c) In a low dose, it has no effect on endothelial cells outside the gut.
    (d) Has been used for pain management in paediatric population.
    (e) Has no side effect in pregnancy and young children.

34. Acetaminophen/paracetamol:
    (a) Is an indirect inhibitor of COX.
    (b) In doses more than 4 grams per day, it may cause liver damage.
    (c) May cause increase in blood pressure and CVS events.
    (d) Is safe in pregnancy.
    (e) Requires N-acetylcysteine for treatment of overdosage.

35. COX inhibitors:
    (a) Paracetamol has good anti-inflammatory action.
    (b) Etoricoxib has shown maximum benefit in arthritis.
    (c) NSAID intake can cause acute renal failure in patients with >10% perioperative blood loss.
    (d) NSAID use can cause congestive heart failure in elderly population.
    (e) Long-term use of proton pump inhibitors used in conjunction with NSAIDs can increase the risk of osteoporotic fractures.

36. COX enzymes:
    (a) Have three independent folding units.
    (b) Both COX-1 and COX-2 are located on chromosome 9.
    (c) TATA box is present in both enzymes.
    (d) COX-2 induction is done by IL-1β.
    (e) COX-2 inhibitors that penetrate blood brain barrier are better analgesics.

37. NSAIDs:
    (a) Effect of NSAIDs is related to its level in affected synovial fluid.
    (b) Renal excretion is the main pathway.
    (c) Haemodialysis leads to increased excretion.
    (d) Aspirin metabolism follows first-order and zero-order kinetics.
    (e) Ketorolac has better efficacy through intranasal route.

38. NSAIDs:
    (a) Unlike other NSAIDs, diclofenac has a higher first-pass metabolism.
    (b) Ibuprofen antagonises the irreversible platelet inhibition induced by aspirin.
    (c) Efficacy of ketoprofen patch is because of lower plasma levels.
    (d) Naproxen is safe in pregnancy.
    (e) Meloxicam should not be used in renal failure.

39. NSAIDs:
    (a) Etoricoxib has significantly less risk of GI events as compared to other NSAIDs.
    (b) Potentiate the effect of warfarin.
    (c) COX-2 inhibitors increase the risk of myocardial infarction.
    (d) Maximum cardiovascular effect is seen with meloxicam.
    (e) COX-2 inhibitors may impair spinal fusion.

40. Tricyclic antidepressants:
    (a) Sodium channel blockade may contribute to its effect.
    (b) Amitriptyline is first-line medication for postherpetic neuralgia.
    (c) Does not have any role in fibromyalgia.
    (d) Selective serotonin reuptake inhibitors may have beneficial effect in fibromyalgia.
    (e) Nausea is a side effect of duloxetine.

41. Calcium channels:
    (a) High voltage-activated calcium channels include L, P/Q and T channels.
    (b) T channels are involved with absence seizures.
    (c) N-type channels are associated with release of neurotransmitter at synaptic junctions.
    (d) P/Q channels are mainly found in the cerebellum.
    (e) L-type channels are only found in skeletal muscle.

42. Gabapentin:
    (a) Binds to $\alpha 2\delta$ subunit of L-type voltage-gated sodium channels.
    (b) Is effective in pain of multiple sclerosis.
    (c) Along with other analgesics in combination, it is more effective in diabetic neuropathy.
    (d) Gastroretentive formulation is more effective in postherpetic neuralgia.
    (e) Enacarbil salt is effective in restless legs syndrome.

43. Pregabalin:
    (a) Works by a similar mechanism as gabapentin.
    (b) Is approved for spinal cord injury pain.
    (c) Has no increased side effect in renal failure.
    (d) Helps in regulating sleep.
    (e) Should be tapered gradually over a 1-week period.

44. Ziconotide:
    (a) Has a peptidic structure.
    (b) Blocks calcium influx into T-type calcium channels.
    (c) Causes early tolerance.
    (d) Is contraindicated in patients with psychosis.
    (e) Has a poor side effect profile.

45. Sodium channels:
    (a) Can cycle open and close rapidly causing seizures.
    (b) Nav1.2 is expressed in sensory neurons.
    (c) Mutations may cause long QT syndrome.
    (d) Have no role in acute pain.
    (e) Phenytoin blocks both fast current and persistent current channels.

46. Sodium channels:
   (a) Are expressed on nociceptive sensory neurons only.
   (b) Mutations lead to decrease in pain.
   (c) Anticonvulsants interact and bind with alpha subunit of channels.
   (d) Mutations can cause migraine.
   (e) Gabapentin only binds to $\delta 1$ and $\delta 2$ fractions.

47. Carbamazepine:
   (a) Is used in postherpetic neuralgia only.
   (b) Side effects can be limited by slow titration.
   (c) Has a lower NNT for trigeminal neuralgia.
   (d) Decreases hyperalgesia in diabetes mellitus.
   (e) Has no major side effect on long-term usage.

48. Lamotrigine:
   (a) Blocks sodium channels in actively firing nerves.
   (b) Increases concentration of glutamate.
   (c) Has a short half-life.
   (d) Has no role in lumbar radicular pain.
   (e) Can be given for all neuropathies.

49. Sodium channels:
   (a) All are expressed on nociceptive sensory neurons.
   (b) Mutations lead to decrease in pain.
   (c) Anticonvulsants interact and bind with α subunit of channel.
   (d) Mutations can cause migraine.
   (e) Gabapentin only binds to $\alpha 2\delta 1$ and $\alpha 2\delta 2$ genes.

50. Anticonvulsants:
   (a) Carbamazepine is the drug of choice for trigeminal neuralgia.
   (b) Oxcarbazepine has no effect on sodium channels.
   (c) Lamotrigine has been effective in HIV neuropathy.
   (d) Lacosamide is a functionalised amino acid.
   (e) Pregabalin has less efficacy than gabapentin.

51. Anticonvulsants:
   (a) Levetiracetam works on sodium channels.
   (b) Retigabine works on potassium channels.

(c) Topiramate acts on multiple receptors.
(d) Valproate acts on multiple receptors.
(e) Perampanel is a selective AMPA-glutamate receptor antagonist.

52. Cannabinoids:
   (a) Work on one receptor only.
   (b) CB1 receptors cause membrane hyperpolarisation and inhibit release of neurotransmitters.
   (c) CB2 receptors causes positive coupling to adenylate cyclase.
   (d) CB1 and CB2 are restricted to neurons only.
   (e) CB1 receptors are present in presynaptic terminals of gabanergic and glutaminergic neurons, Aδ and C fibres.

53. Endocannabinoids:
   (a) Anandamide is the only preparation known.
   (b) Synthesis is seen in neurons.
   (c) Anandamide causes inhibition of adenyl cyclase to cause effect.
   (d) Anandamide is degraded by fatty acid amide hydrolase (FAAH).
   (e) 2-AG is a full agonist at CB1 receptors.

54. α2 agonists:
   (a) Can cause sedation and vasodepression when given in analgesic doses.
   (b) Tizanidine is effective in myofascial and neuropathic pain.
   (c) Mechanism of action involves activation of postsynaptic receptors.
   (d) Activation leads to analgesic properties.
   (e) Adrenoceptor agonism is responsible for action of clonidine.

55. NMDA receptors:
   (a) Cause analgesic reaction by blockade of glutamate action.
   (b) Ketamine supresses central sensitisation.
   (c) Agents acting on glycine co-agonist site on the NMDA receptor complex may have less side effects.
   (d) Methadone is the only opioid drug to have actions at NMDA receptors.
   (e) Memantine is effective in diabetic neuropathy.

56. Skeletal muscle relaxants:
   (a) Cause depression of postsynaptic reflexes within the dorsal horn.
   (b) Cyclobenzaprine has no drug interactions.

(c) Orphenadrine is contraindicated in neuromuscular junction defects.
(d) Diazepam works with GABA-mediated presynaptic inhibition.
(e) Baclofen can be administered intrathecally.

✅ **Answers**

1. T F T T T

   GPCR contain seven hydrophobic transmembrane domains interconnected by short loops and display an extracellular N-terminal domain and an intracellular C-terminal tail. Mu, delta and kappa are highly homologous with transmembrane domains and intracellular loops alike. The extracellular loops and N and C tails differ and are important for respective selectivity.

2. T F T T T

   Opioid receptor signalling involves inhibition of calcium channels or activation of potassium channels. It also involves inhibition of cAMP. Signalling involves G protein-independent pathways via beta-arrestins which are a family of proteins important for regulating signal transduction at G protein-coupled receptors. Delta receptors are committed to lysosomal degeneration.

3. T F T T T

   Kappa receptor-mediated analgesia is independent from mu and delta receptor-mediated analgesia especially in thermal pain. Spinal analgesia is mediated by mu receptors, while supraspinal analgesia is mediated by both mu and delta receptors. Nortriptyline is a tricyclic antidepressant that reverses mechanical allodynia of neuropathic pain. Prodynorphin controls nociceptive responses from dual opioid (kappa) and nonopioid activities (NMDA).

4. T F T T F

   Opioid receptors are mostly located in laminae I and II. Opioid binding is maxim with mu (70%), delta (24%) and kappa receptors (6%). Opioid receptors are mainly on fine (Aδ and C fibre-mediated noxious and static allodynia) afferent terminals, so Aβ fibres (mediating dynamic allodynia) are mostly not affected by opioids.

5. T T F T T

   Main sites for action are periaqueductal grey area and rostral ventromedial area. Fibres descending from PAG are mainly GABAergic but also serotonergic, enchpelargic and glycinergic. Tapentadol causes analgesia via inhibitory α2 adrenoreceptors. Tramadol is a dual serotonin and nor-adrenaline uptake inhibitor.

6. T T F T T
    Dynamic allodynia is difficult to assess while static can be evoked by increased pressure on the skin. Dynamic mechanical allodynia is sig-nalled by large diameter myelinated Aβ sensory neurons. Morphine is effective only when given systematically in diabetes neuropathy. Nerve injury leads to reduced presynaptic opioid receptors and changes in cal-cium channels resulting in increased transmitter release.

7. T F F T T
    Codeine is metabolised in liver by glucuronidation, N-demethylation and O-demethylation. Demethylation converts it into morphine. It is inferior to ibuprofen and diclofenac in analgesic efficacy. Codeine brings NNT of 1 gram of paracetamol from 3.8 to 2.2 when used in conjunction.

8. T T T F T
    NNT of tramadol varies with the dosage (50 mg, 8.5; 75 mg, 5.3; 100 mg, 4.8; 150 mg, 2.9). Tramadol has good efficacy in fibromyalgia. Risk of addiction is 1:100,000.

9. T T T T T
    Bioavailability is less because of higher first-pass metabolism. Active metabolites are morphine 6 glucuronide and morphine 3 glucuronide, and both can cause neurotoxicity. Morphine 6 glucuronide gets accumulated in renal failure and can cause respiratory depression. Morphine 3 glucuronide may produce side effects that may oppose morphine's actions – allodynia, hyperalgesia, myoclonus and seizures.

10. T F T F T
    Bioavailability of oxycodone is more than morphine (>60%). Oxycodone is also effective for visceral pain as it has agonistic effect on kappa receptors. Oxycodone has potent effect on mu receptors but also good effect on kappa receptors; thus it is an ideal medication for opioid rotation.

11. T F T F T
    Methadone has good oral bioavailability, high potency and long duration of action. The mechanism of action involves mu and delta agonism, NMDA antagonism and serotonin reuptake blockade.

12. T T T F T

Methadone is a mix of D and L isomer. L isomer is responsible for its opioid receptor affinity. The half-life is 27 h because of lipophilicity and extensive tissue distribution. Gut acidity can increase absorption while alkaline urine (pH > 6) can decrease clearance from 30% to almost nil (oral bioavailability of opioids: methadone, 80%; tramadol, 80%; codeine, 60%; oxycodone, 60%; morphine, 30%).

13. F T F F T

It is ideal for transmucosal and transdermal administration because of high lipid solubility, low molecular weight and high potency. Systemic levels are up to 90% after transdermal administration. Steady-state concentration is reached in 6 days, and after removal of the patch, 16 h is required for the systemic levels to come down to 50%.

14. T T T T T

Bioavailability of fentanyl is 51%, methadone is 34% and morphine is 18%. Iontophoresis is a modification of transdermal administration of drugs that is achieved by applying electric current to deliver drugs in an ionised state. Subcutaneous administration rate should not exceed 5 l/h to avoid patient discomfort.

15. F T T T T

Tolerance to respiratory depression occurs rapidly and is irreversible. Buprenorphine and tramadol have less respiratory depression. Tolerance to sedation develops over a period of 1 week.

16. T T T F T

Occurrence of withdrawal symptoms after abrupt discontinuation may be seen in the form of yawning, diaphoresis, lacrimation and tachycardia. Intramuscular route is not reliable because of slow and unpredictable absorption.

17. T F F T F

Opioid receptors are also located on dorsal root ganglia and peripheral nerves. Opioid receptors are present at both presynaptic and postsynaptic sites. Mu receptors modulate input from mechanical, chemical and thermal stimuli. Kappa receptors influence thermal stimuli and chemical visceral pain, while delta receptors modulate mechanical and inflammatory pain. Opioids undergo hepatic metabolism via uridine diphosphate glucuronosyltransferase enzymes by adding glucuronic acid moiety.

Metabolites are excreted in urine, bile and faeces (especially methadone). CYP-2D6 is not present in 10% of white population and thus making them poor metabolisers.

18. F T T F T

Morphine takes 24 h to achieve steady-state concentration, while methadone takes 7 days for the same. Methadone is useful in short gut syndrome as it has intrinsically longer plasma life. Constipation due to opioids is seen due to decreased gastric motility due to binding of opioid receptors in the antrum of stomach and proximal part of small bowel. The primary mechanism is gut immotility, so treatment includes active laxative like senna, lactulose or bisacodyl.

19. T T T T T

Nalbuphine (mu receptor antagonist and kappa receptor agonist) reduces the itching. Histamine activates C fibre itch receptors and causes itching in the face and perineum region. Naloxone can precipitate congestive heart failure in patients on opioids for more than 1 week.

20. T F F T T

Opioids decrease immunologic function via its effect on antibody and cellular immune responses, NK cell activity, cytokine expression and phagocytic activity. Females also suffer from sexual dysfunction in the form of dysmenorrhoea. Opioids cause GABA signalling via inhibition of acetylcholine release in the medial pontine reticular formation in the primary focus of disruption of sleep.

21. T T T F T

Withdrawal symptoms last for 3–7 days. Clonidine is an alpha2 agonist, and 0.2–0.4 mg/day helps in weaning from opioids.

22. F T F T T

Codeine is similar in structure to morphine but affinity is 300 times less. Codeine is mainly metabolised by uridine diphosphate, while only 3% conversion is because of CYP2D6.

23. T T T F T

Acetaminophen works by prostaglandin inhibition along with inhibition of PG endoperoxide H2 synthase and COX centrally. The metabolism is mainly in the liver (90%) via glucuronidation and sulphate conjugation. Ten percent undergoes oxidative metabolism via CYP system. Toxicity is

increased with low glutathione levels as seen in chronic hepatitis c, mal-
nourishment, HIV infection and cirrhosis.

24. T F T T T
Alcohol usage contributes to drug-induced hepatotoxicity via induction
of CYP2E1 and NAPQ1 formation.

25. T F T F F
Tramadol is a synthetic racemic mixture and is a weak opioid with mild
serotonin and norepinephrine reuptake properties. Tramadol is par-
tially antagonised by naloxone. It also acts on alpha 2 receptors.
Extended release tramadol reaches steady state in 4 days. Maximum
bioavailability is seen via oral route (100%), followed by rectal route
(78%). It is excreted mainly via the kidneys (90%) and also in faeces
(10%). Extended release formulation causes side effects only in 6% of
patients. The side effects include dizziness, fatigue, sweating, dry
mouth, drowsiness, sedation and orthostatic hypotension. Serotonin
toxicity occurs because of overstimulation of 5HT1A and 5HT2 receptors in the brain.

26. T T F T T
Steroids cause decrease in cancer pain by inhibition of prostaglandin synthesis and reduction in peritumour and perineural oedema. The main side
effect is weight gain (70%) followed by skin bruising (53%), sleep disturbances (45%), mood symptoms (42%) and fractures (12%). Low-dose steroid therapy has a role in chemotherapy-induced peripheral neuropathy.
Disc disruption causes release of pro-inflammatory mediators and neuro-
sensitising chemicals which are attenuated by steroids.

27. T T T F F
NNT of topical steroids for acute pain is 3.9 and for chronic pain is 3.1.
TRPV1 receptors are also activated by heat >43 degrees, decreased pH
and bradykinin. TRPV2 is activated by heat (>52 degrees). Menthol provides analgesia by calcium and kappa-opioid receptors.

28. T F T T T

29. T F T T F
Prostaglandin formation is a two-step process with an initial COX reaction and second hydroxyperoxidase reaction. COX-1 is expressed in most
tissues, whereas COX-2 is expressed on inflammatory stimuli especially in

macrophages. COX-2 expression is seen in endothelial cells and in kidneys and inhibition may cause side effects. COX-3 results from alternative splicing of COX-1 gene and retention of intron 1. It has been only detected in dogs.

30. T T T T T

Prostaglandins E2 and I2 (prostacyclin) increase sensitivity of peripheral nociceptor endings and facilitate activation of nociceptive transduction processes such as TRPV1 and voltage-gated sodium channel (Nav1.8). Application of PGE2 to isolated dorsal root ganglion increases current response to heat and capsaicin. Modulation of sodium channels involves activation of adenyl cyclise and increase in cAMP which leads to protein kinase A-dependent phosphorylation of the channels. Inhibition of platelet aggregation occurs through reduced formation of COX-1-dependent thromboxane in platelets.

31. T T T T T

COX-2 metabolises the endocannabinoids arachidonoylglycerol. Flurbiprofen also increases spinal endocannabinoids. Aspirin-triggered lipoxins are formed by aspirin/acetylsalicylic acid. S enantiomer is a direct COX inhibitor.

32. F F T F T

Diclofenac acts mainly on COX-2. Galenic formulation of diclofenac contains monolithic acid-resistant encapsulation and can stay in the stomach for hours to days. Diclofenac has significant first-pass metabolism, and hence the bioavailability is only 50%. High first-pass metabolism also leads to reactive metabolites leading to liver toxicity. Postoperative bleeding seen with ketorolac is because of long inhibition of COX-1.

33. T F T T F

Aspirin acetylates a serine residue in the active centre of COX-1 and COX-2. Aspirin blocks COX-1 irreversibly, and the body's thromboxane synthesis is affected for few days. Low-dose aspirin does not affect prostacyclin synthesis, and antithrombotic activity is maintained. Aspirin has been used in Kawasaki syndrome and acute rheumatic fever. In pregnancy it may cause premature bleeding and before puberty may cause Reye's syndrome with liver and brain damage.

34. T T T T T

   If used in pregnancy, it may cause cryptorchidism in male offspring.

35. F T T T T

   Paracetamol is a COX inhibitor in the brain and has no effect on peripheral COX thus not having any anti-inflammatory actions. Etoricoxib in a dose of 60–90 mg has a NNT of 7 or 8 for at least 50% pain relief over a 12-week period.

36. T F F T T

   Independent folding units are epidermal growth factor-like domain, membrane-binding moiety and active enzymatic domain. COX-1 is located on chromosome 9 and COX-2 on chromosome 1. TATA box is a DNA sequence that indicates where a genetic sequence can be read and decoded. It is a type of promoter sequence which specifies to other molecules where transcription begins. Pro-inflammatory cytokine IL-1β is upregulated at the site of inflammation and plays a role in activation of COX-2 in periphery and brain.

37. T F F T T

   NSAIDs are highly bound to plasma proteins and thus not removed by haemodialysis. Ketorolac has advantage of blood-brain barrier penetration via olfactory route with minimal GI effects.

38. T T T F T

   High first-pass metabolism leads to lower bioavailability. High tissue concentrations are seen as a result of patch which means more therapeutic effect, but low plasma concentrations mean systemic adverse effects. Naproxen can cross placenta and cause neonatal jaundice.

39. T T T F T

   Etoricoxib has 40% less risk of GI events. NSAIDs potentiate the effect of warfarin by displacing protein-bound drug or by inhibiting its metabolism by hepatic microsomal enzymes. COX-2 inhibitors only decrease production of PGI2 without affecting thromboxane A2 synthesis. Cardiovascular risk is significant with rofecoxib (45%), followed by diclofenac (40%), indomethacin (30%) and meloxicam (20%). COX-2 inhibitors impair spinal fusion by inhibition of inflammatory processes with a concomitant reduction in blood flow in the early period of osteogenesis, decreased mesenchymal cell proliferation or inhibition of calcification of bone matrix.

40. T T F T T
Amitriptyline is the most potent followed by doxepin and imipramine. Neural blockade with amitriptyline is use dependent. TCAs have positive effect on sleep, fatigue, pain and well-being but not on trigger points. Fluoxetine at doses of 45 g/day had significant improvement in Fibromyalgia Impact Questionnaire. Duloxetine is a serotonergic and nor-adrenergic reuptake inhibitor. Nausea is self-limiting.

41. F T T T F
High-voltage channels include L, P/Q and R channels. T is a low-voltage channel. T channels regulate firing by participating in bursting and intrinsic oscillations and are associated with absence seizures. P/Q channels were first described in Purkinje cells and hence the name. L-type channels are also found in neuronal and smooth muscle.

42. T T T T T
Binding to $\alpha2\delta$ subunit decreases release of glutamate, norepinephrine and substance P. It is effective in multiple sclerosis especially with a throbbing, pricking and cramping quality. Gabapentin and nortriptyline in combination are highly effective in diabetic neuropathy.

43. T T F T T
The dosage should be reduced in renal failure. Sudden discontinuation can cause insomnia, nausea, headache and diarrhoea.

44. T F F T T
It is a ω-conopeptide and because of peptidic structure it can be administered intrathecally. It blocks N-type calcium channels in dorsal horn laminae of the spinal cord. It does not cause tolerance, dependence and respiratory depression. Side effects include dizziness, ataxia, confusion and headache. If given in psychosis, it can cause hallucinations.

45. T F T T T
Sensory neurons express Na1.2, Na1.8 and Na1.9. Na1.7 is in peripheral nervous system along with Na1.4 and Na1.5 in muscles. Mutations in Na 1.5 cause long QT syndrome, while mutations in Na1.4 cause hypercalcaemic

periodic paralysis. Persistent sodium current is a small fraction of the fast current and has a role in regulating excitability.

46. F F T T T

Na1.1, 1.3 and 1.6 are seen on neuronal cell bodies and dendrites. Na1.2 and 1.6 are seen on axons, especially Na1.6 on nodes of Ranvier. Na1.6, 1.7, 1.8 and 1.9 are seen on nociceptive sensory neurons. Mutations of sodium channels may cause inherited erythromelalgia (intense pain, erythema, burning sensation and swelling of limbs), paroxysmal extreme pain disorder (severe rectal, ocular and mandibular pain). Nav1.1 mutation may lead to familial hemiplegic migraine.

47. F T T T F

It is also used in diabetic neuropathy, post-stroke pain and Guillain-Barré syndrome. Side effects include drowsiness, dizziness, nausea, vomiting, pancytopenia and Stevens-Johnson syndrome. Long-term usage causes agranulocytosis and aplastic anaemia.

48. T F F F F

It decreases concentration of glutamate which is an excitatory neurotransmitter. It is 55% bound to proteins and has a half-life of about 30 h. Higher doses are effective in radicular pain (400 mg/day). It does not have any role in HIV neuropathy.

49. F F T T T

Nav1.1, 1.3, and 1.6 are seen on neuronal cell bodies and dendrites. Nav1.2 and 1.6 are seen on axons. Nav1.6 is seen on nodes of Ranvier. Nav1.6, 1.7, 1.8 and 1.9 are seen on nociceptive sensory neurons. Mutations cause increase in pain. Inherited erythromelalgia is seen which manifests as intense pain, erythema, burning sensation and swelling of limbs. Paroxysmal extreme pain disorder manifests as severe rectal, ocular and mandibular pain. Nav1.1 mutation can cause familial hemiplegic migraine.

50. T F T T F

Oxcarbazepine works by blockade of voltage-gated sodium channels, inhibition of high threshold calcium channels and enhancement of potassium rectifier. Pregabalin is more potent in binding affinity than gabapentin, has more than 90% bioavailability and exhibits liver pharmacokinetics.

51. F T T T T
Levetiracetam modulates release of neurotransmitter by binding to vesi-
cle protein SV2. The most important side effect of retigabine is urinary
retention. Topiramate acts on sodium, calcium, GABAa and AMPA/kainate
receptors.

52. F T F F T
CB1, CB2 and GPR55 activate increased calcium and M currents which
engages signalling mechanisms distinct from CB1 and CB2. CB2 receptors
cause negative coupling to adenylate cyclase via Gi/o and activation of
extracellular signal-regulated kinase and voltage-dependent calcium
channels. CB1 is restricted to neurons, and expression is high at several
important loci in the brain, spinal cord and peripheral nervous system.
CB2 are restricted to cells of immune system especially glia. Twenty-five
percent of cells of dorsal root ganglion express CB1.

53. F F F T T
The other members of the family are 2-arachidonoylglycerol, noladin
ether and virodhamine. The synthesis is in neurons apart from basophils,
macrophages and microglia. Anandamide also causes inhibition of N-P/Q
and L-type voltage-gated calcium channels. Ibuprofen and ketorolac
inhibit FAAH.

54. T T T T T
A2 receptors are coupled to increase outward potassium conductance
which reduces cellular excitability.

55. T T T F T
Methadone has effect on NMDA receptors along with dextropropoxyphene
and pethidine.

56. T F T T T
Muscle-relaxing effect is seen because of inhibition of interneuronal activity
and blocking of polysynaptic neurons in the spinal cord and descending
reticular formation. Cyclobenzaprine when administered with tramadol can
cause seizures. Coadministration with monoamine oxidase inhibitors is contraindicated. Orphenadrine is a direct descendant of diphenhydramine and
exhibits anticholinergic and antihistaminic properties.

Non-pharmacological Interventions

? Questions

1. Psychological aspects of chronic pain:
   (a) High motivation towards achievement in childhood is a risk factor for pain-prone personalities.
   (b) Is mostly associated with inconsistent report of person's pain with anatomic distribution.
   (c) Pain behaviour can be acquired by observing other people's reactions to pain.
   (d) Both overt and covert coping mechanisms help gain control over the pain.
   (e) Adapting coping strategies can help in treating chronic pain.

2. Cognitive behavioural therapy (CBT):
   (a) Cognitive behavioural perspective is same as therapy.
   (b) Four key components help gain more control over pain.
   (c) Cognitive restructuring involves identifying maladaptive thoughts and achieving control of affect.
   (d) CBT has no role in restoring mood.
   (e) Role playing skills can help in managing pain.

3. Psychologic interventions:
   (a) Biofeedback has no role in visceral pain.
   (b) Biofeedback has no role in headache.
   (c) Biofeedback involves dysregulation of autonomic nervous system.
   (d) Mindfulness meditation is same as transcendental meditation.
   (e) Long-term meditation can increase cortical thickness.

4. Cognitive behavioural therapy (CBT):
   (a) Has six phases.
   (b) Works mainly on the premise of changing patient's thinking and behaviour from well-established ineffective responses.
   (c) Stress is a major component of physical symptoms in elderly.
   (d) Distraction is one of the coping mechanisms.
   (e) Catastrophising helps in coping.

5. Physical medicine techniques:
   (a) Physical and occupational therapists provide the same input.
   (b) Involve a mix of cognitive behavioural approach plus intensive physical training.
   (c) Functional capacity evaluation has been shown to predict return to work.

(d) Electromyography can ascertain if disc bulges can produce nerve damage.

(e) Specificity of EMG in diagnosing radiculopathy is more than MRI scan.

6. Physical modalities in treatment of pain:
   (a) Heat exerts its effect on peripheral levels.
   (b) Warm water hydrotherapy provides heat by convection.
   (c) Heat therapy has no role in sympathetic-mediated pain.
   (d) Ultrasound is more useful at muscle-bone interface.
   (e) Laminectomy site is a contraindication for ultrasound treatment.

7. Mind-body medicine:
   (a) Is based on the assertion that the mind can positively affect the body.
   (b) Relaxation can help break pain cycle.
   (c) Can decrease the perception of pain.
   (d) Relaxation works through the normalisation of stress hormones.
   (e) Yoga is the only effective technique.

8. Mind-body medicine:
   (a) Guided imagery has benefit only in fibromyalgia.
   (b) Hypnosis works by decreasing anxiety and depression.
   (c) Iyengar yoga reduces pain intensity, functional disability and depression.
   (d) Tai chi and qigong can increase bone density.
   (e) Music therapy has shown benefit in decreasing anxiety.

9. Mind-body medicine:
   (a) Massage has no dangerous side effects.
   (b) Chiropractic is based mainly on high-velocity, low-amplitude thrust manipulation.
   (c) Osteopathic manipulation is effective in neck and head pain.
   (d) Glucosamine and chondroitin have efficacy in osteoarthritis.
   (e) S-adenosylmethionine has anti-inflammatory and analgesic effects.

10. Acupuncture:
    (a) Is based on theory of yin and yang.
    (b) Meridians are defined by physical structures.
    (c) Needles produced analgesia by extremely painful stimuli.
    (d) Has units which are in relation to patient's own body.
    (e) Works on gate control theory.

11. Acupuncture:
    (a) 2 Hz stimulation selectively accelerates release of encephalin.
    (b) Effects can be reversed by selective serotonin reuptake inhibitors.
    (c) Pneumothorax is the main side effect.
    (d) Sham acupuncture provides a true placebo effect.
    (e) Most useful in postoperative pain.

12. Acupuncture
    (a) Can decrease postoperative opioid requirements.
    (b) Magnets can be used to provide acupuncture.
    (c) Neck mobility is increased.
    (d) Decreases median nerve sensory latency in carpal tunnel syndrome.
    (e) Has no role in neuropathic pain.

13. Opioids as neuraxial agents:
    (a) Act on postsynaptic receptors only.
    (b) Onset of analgesia is quick by intrathecal route than epidural route.
    (c) Mode of action of fentanyl is same via both epidural or via continuous route.
    (d) Hydrophilic opioids have more rostral spread.
    (e) Are very effective in neuropathic pain.

14. Intrathecal calcium channel antagonists:
    (a) Mostly involves N-type channels.
    (b) Ziconotide blocks N-type channels.
    (c) Tolerance is the main problem.
    (d) Side effects include confusion, somnolence and urinary retention.
    (e) Intrathecal verapamil decreases postoperative analgesic requirements.

15. Intrathecal GABA agonists:
    (a) All GABA receptors are ligand-gated ion channels.
    (b) Both GABA receptors work by different mechanisms.
    (c) GABAβ receptor agonists produce post- and presynaptic inhibition.
    (d) Intrathecal effect is only produced by GABAβ agonists.
    (e) Both GABAα and GABAβ agonists produce motor blockade.

16. Intrathecal adrenergic agonists:
    (a) Causes analgesia via α1 and α2 receptors.
    (b) α2 Agonists increase C fibre release.

(c) Dexmedetomidine has better clinical profile.

(d) Cannot be used in paediatric patient.

(e) Side effects of α2 agonists are because of effect on preganglionic fibres in the thoracic spinal cord.

17. Intrathecal glutaminergic receptor antagonists:
    (a) Are either G protein-coupled or ion channel receptors.
    (b) Ketamine is a non-competitive NMDA antagonist.
    (c) S enantiomer of ketamine produces long-lasting pain relief.
    (d) Focal lymphocytic vasculitis at site of catheter insertion is a side effect.
    (e) S enantiomer causes histologic changes in the spinal cord.

18. Dorsal rhizotomy and ganglionectomy:
    (a) Selectively interrupts sensory transmission without injuring motor pathways.
    (b) Neuroma formation is a risk factor.
    (c) Ganglionectomy may lead to Wallerian degeneration.
    (d) Ganglionectomy has shown good results in thoracic and occipital pain.
    (e) Dorsal rhizotomy is performed through intradural approach, whereas ganglionectomy is performed extradurally.

19. Dorsal root entry zone ablation:
    (a) Dorsal root entry zone comprises of Lissauer's tract and Rexed's layers I–V.
    (b) During ablation, best location for ablation is determined where stimulation elicits maximum response in DREZ.
    (c) 1–2 lesions are required per avulsed root.
    (d) Pain relief remains the same after ablation.
    (e) Complications include sensory ataxia, motor deficits, dysesthesias and myelopathy.

20. Cordotomy:
    (a) Anterolateral cordotomy aims at lateral spinothalamic tract.
    (b) Is mostly used in malignancy.
    (c) Is very effective for the burning component of the neuropathic pain.
    (d) Lesioning is done at 35 mA (60–75°) with up to a maximum of 50 mA (90°).
    (e) Associated with high incidence of death.

21. Spinal cord stimulation:
    (a) Applied in dorsal horn activates fibres in both directions.
    (b) Mainly works by GABA receptors.
    (c) Cholinergic activation decreases the response to spinal cord stimulation.
    (d) Works by resolution of tissue ischaemia in ischaemic extremity pain.
    (e) Preemptive stimulation may be protective in angina.

22. Spinal cord stimulation:
    (a) R-III reflex in QST has sensitivity to the outcome of SCS.
    (b) Trial period is not preferred for angina pectoris.
    (c) Has no benefit in postherpetic neuralgia.
    (d) Use of 16 polar electrode lead can produce paraesthesias.
    (e) Helps reduce phantom sensation more than the phantom pain.

✅ Answers

1. T T T T T
    Risk factors for pain-prone personalities include high motivation towards achievement, emotional abuse, family dysfunction, illness or death of a parent and responsibilities early in life. Overt coping mechanisms include rest, meditation and relaxation. Covert mechanisms include distraction, problem-solving and seeking information.

2. F T T F T
    Cognitive behavioural perspective is patient's perspective that they are helpless because of the pain. CBT approach combines cognitive and behavioural techniques. Four key components are education, skills education, skills consolidation, generalisation and maintenance. CBT restores function and mood and reduces pain- and disability-related behaviour.

3. F F T F T
    Biofeedback has a role in back pain and chronic myofascial pain and has shown efficacy in irritable bowel syndrome. Electromyographic feedback in tension headache helps in relaxing frontalis muscle. Patients with migraine are provided with thermal feedback. Biofeedback decreases nociceptive stimuli from autonomic nervous system. Transcendental meditation focuses more on one of the senses, whereas mindfulness is opposite and goal is awareness of whole perceptual field. Long-term

meditation can increase cortical thickness especially in areas of somato-sensory, auditory, visual and interoceptive processing.

4. T T F T F

    The phases of CBT are initial assessment, collaborative acquisition of skills, consolidation of skills, generalisation, maintenance and relapse prevention, booster sessions and follow-up. Other coping mechanisms are reassuring and seeking information. Catastrophising is an important factor in poor coping. It is engaging in negative thoughts about one's plight.

5. F T F T T

    Physical therapists focus on the strength, flexibility and coordination of large muscle groups, whereas occupational therapists focus on fine and gross motor strength, flexibility and coordination of the hands and activities of daily life. Physical training includes aerobic capacity, muscle strength, endurance and coordination. Functional capacity evaluation is helpful in charting changes in function, identifying non-medical factors influencing the ability to work. Electromyography also can help in diagnosing spinal stenosis but does not predict future pain. Electromyography not only tells which nerve is involved but also severity and chronicity of lesion.

6. F T F T T

    Heat exerts its effect on spinal and supraspinal levels. Superficial modalities include hot packs, heating pads and heat lamps, while deep heating agents include ultrasound, short wave and microwave. CRPS can be helped with fluidotherapy which uses glass beads and pulverised corn cobs that have low heat affinity and are heated by hot air. Energy is absorbed more effectively in ultrasound resulting in higher tissue temperatures. Contraindications for ultrasound treatment are laminectomy site, metal pacemakers, spinal cord stimulators, surgical implants and copper-containing intrauterine devices because of risk of excessive heating.

7. T T T T F

    Relaxation works through normalisation of cortisol, epinephrine and nor-epinephrine. Mind-body medicine techniques include yoga, abdominal breathing, meditation, guided imagery, biofeedback and tai chi.

8. F T T T T

Guided imagery is the generation of specific mental images to evolve a state of relaxation or physiologic change. It is beneficial in fibromyalgia, tension headache and recurrent abdominal pain. Iyengar yoga has emphasis on detail, precision and alignment in the performance of posture and breath control. Tai chi and qigong are ancient meditative movement techniques that combine physical movements with meditation and relaxation. Music therapy decreases anxiety in ventilated patients, especially after open heart surgery and colonoscopy.

9. F T T T T

Massage is contraindicated in metastatic lesions, severe osteoporosis, thrombosis, infection and bleeding disorders. Both glucosamine and chondroitin are ω-3 fatty acids useful in rheumatoid arthritis.

10. T F F T T

Yang is related to bright, hot, activity, dry and male, whereas yin is dark, wet and female. Acupuncture is based on promoting balance between yang and yin. Meridians are not defined by physical structures but are defined by their function through which energy (Qi) flows). Needle twirling produces heavy or numb sensation (de qi). Tsun represents a distance equal to the space between the distal and interphalangeal joint and proximal interphalangeal joint on the middle finger. Acupuncture acts by stimulating Aβ fibres and inhibits spinal transmission of pain by smaller Aδ and C fibres.

11. F F F F T

2 Hz stimulation releases enkephalins, β-endorphins and endomorphin, whereas 100 Hz stimulation increases the release of dynorphin only. Maximum effect is achieved by stimulating both frequencies. Effects can be reversed by naloxone and SSRIs. Main complications are bleeding, needle pain and pneumothorax. Meridians cover the entire body, and hence sham acupuncture still provides some effect.

12. T T T T F

Postoperative morphine requirements are observed to decrease by 50%. Acupuncture has shown some benefit in HIV neuropathy.

13. F F F T F

Opioids act on postsynaptic receptors located on cells originating in the dorsal horn but also on presynaptic receptors found on spinal terminals of primary afferent fibres. Onset of analgesia is same via both the routes. Fentanyl acts mostly via spinal route if given via epidural route, whereas if given as continuous infusion, uptake via systemic absorption plays a role. Hydrophilic opioids have more rostral spread as compared to lipophilic opioids, and that is the reason they have more spread into the brain. Tactile allodynia seen in neuropathic pain is less responsive.

14. T T F T T

Other channels involved are N, P/Q and L type. Intrathecal gabapentin exerts its effects on same channels. Ziconotide is a synthetic form of peptide, ω-conotoxin MVIIA, isolated from the venom of marine cone snail *Conus magus*. Tolerance never happens with calcium channel receptors. Only 30% experience serious side effects.

15. F T T F F

GABAα is ligand-gated ion receptor, whereas GABAβ is a metabotropic receptor. GABAα causes influx of chloride channels and stabilisation of membrane potential which decreases neuronal excitability. GABAβ causes activation of inwardly rectifying potassium channels, inhibition of calcium channels and inhibition of adenylate cyclase. Baclofen blocks the release of glutamate, substance P and CGRP. Neither of the agonists produce motor blockade.

16. F F T F T

Intrathecal agents only act via $\alpha 2$ receptors. $\alpha 1$ receptors are present on smooth muscle cells of peripheral vasculature. $\alpha 2$ receptors are present in CNS/PNS which modulates pain signal. Clonidine decreases presynaptic C fibre transmitter release and hyperpolarises the postsynaptic membrane. Dexmedetomidine has better analgesia with less side effects. Intrathecal agents have good analgesic effect in neuropathic pain and cancer pain in paediatric population.

17. T T T T T

18. T F T T T

Neuroma formation is not common as distal afferent fibres remain intact in the case of rhizotomy and degenerate following ganglionectomy. Wallerian degeneration of peripheral afferents may occur along with target tissue denervation leading to pain and dysesthesias. Ganglionectomy has shown good effect in 68% of population for thoracic pain and up to 80% for occipital neuralgia.

19. T F F F T

    During ablation, location is ascertained where stimulation elicits no response. 20–30 lesions are required per avulsed root. Amount of pain relief decreases with time.

20. T T F T F

    Anterolateral cordotomy aims at spinothalamic tract and thus interrupts pain signals from opposite side of body below the level of the lesion. The main indication is unilateral nociceptive pain secondary to malignancy. Cordotomy relives stimulus-evoked hyperpathia in intractable neuropathic pain with no effect on burning component. The main complications are transient weakness (4–17%), ataxia (4%), death (3%) and hypotension (2%).

21. T T F T T

    Dorsal horn application activates fibres both orthodromically and anti-dromically. GABA receptor agonism may increase the response to spinal cord stimulation. It increases blood flow and decreases oxygen tissue demand. It also increases peripheral release of CGRP which causes vaso-dilation. Preemptive stimulation makes the heart more resistant to critical ischaemia.

22. T T F T T

    Normally the trial period is at least 1 week.

Neuropathic Pain

© Springer International Publishing AG 2018
R. Gupta, *Multiple Choice Questions in Pain Management*,
DOI 10.1007/978-3-319-56917-8_5

❓ Questions

1. Postherpetic neuralgia:
   (a) Varicella reactivation is necessary for PHN.
   (b) Seen in less than 10% of patients more than 85 years old with defects in cell-mediated immunity.
   (c) Female gender is a risk factor.
   (d) Most common site of involvement is the thoracic region.
   (e) Administration of zoster vaccine results in an extreme reduction of herpes zoster and postherpetic neuralgia.

2. Postherpetic neuralgia:
   (a) After initial infection, virus remains latent in sensory nerve ganglia of trigeminal or thoracic ganglia.
   (b) Rash is mostly bilateral.
   (c) Inflammatory changes are caused by virus.
   (d) Two main mechanisms for pain are sensitisation and deafferentation.
   (e) Hyperalgesia is seen with allodynia in the absence of sensory changes.

3. Postherpetic neuralgia:
   (a) Mostly a purpuric rash is seen.
   (b) Mostly resolves in about 6 months.
   (c) Antiretroviral medications are not effective.
   (d) Topical lidocaine is ineffective.
   (e) Capsaicin works by desensitisation of nerve root endings.

4. Treatment of postherpetic neuralgia:
   (a) Pregabalin is better tolerated because of better bioavailability.
   (b) Venlafaxine is effective at dosages <200 mg/day.
   (c) Opioids are not effective in management.
   (d) Intrathecal methylprednisolone is effective.
   (e) There is no role for spinal cord stimulation.

5. Diabetic neuropathy:
   (a) Only sensory neuropathy is seen.
   (b) Pain is seen in 20% of patients.
   (c) Neuropathic pain is seen more in type 2 diabetes than type 1.
   (d) Arterial hypertension is a risk factor.
   (e) Ion channel dysfunction is mainly responsible for neuropathy.

6. Diabetic neuropathy:
   (a) Polyol pathway prevents damage.
   (b) Neuronal ischaemia and infarction are also seen.
   (c) Chronic hyperglycaemia leads to decrease in nerve conduction.
   (d) NADPH is protective against oxidative stress.
   (e) Altered calcium and sodium channels dysfunction contributes to injury.

7. Diabetic neuropathy:
   (a) Most common is chronic sensorimotor peripheral neuropathy.
   (b) Most commonly hands are involved.
   (c) Large nerve fibres are involved.
   (d) Loss of proprioception and vibration is an early finding.
   (e) Gait ataxia may be seen.

8. Diabetic neuropathy:
   (a) Morton's neuroma is a differential diagnosis.
   (b) Autonomic neuropathy is only seen in type 1 diabetes mellitus.
   (c) Both myelinated and unmyelinated nerves are affected.
   (d) Can cause osteoporosis.
   (e) Diabetic amyotrophy is seen in both type 1 and type 2 diabetes.

9. Diabetic neuropathy:
   (a) Mononeuropathies mostly involve cranial nerves.
   (b) Most effective treatment is anticonvulsants.
   (c) Gabapentin has better clinical profile than pregabalin.
   (d) Duloxetine has no effect.
   (e) Tramadol helps with allodynia and paraesthesia.

10. Diabetic neuropathy:
    (a) Mononeuropathies are commonly seen.
    (b) Third nerve palsy is rarely seen.
    (c) Mononeuropathies show vascular occlusion.
    (d) Main change seen is demyelination.
    (e) Diabetic amyotrophy is not painful.

11. HIV-related neuropathy:
    (a) Is the most common neurologic abnormality seen.
    (b) Is seen in 90% of HIV infection.

(c) Sensory neuropathy is mainly seen.

(d) CD4 count <50 cells/mm is a risk factor.

(e) Painful dysesthesia, allodynia and hyperalgesia are seen.

12. HIV-related neuropathy:

(a) Mostly lower extremities are involved.

(b) Numbness is the initial symptom.

(c) Reflexes are not lost.

(d) Mostly small fibre neuropathy is seen.

(e) Dorsal root ganglion loss is more than distal axon loss.

13. HIV-related neuropathy:

(a) Is cytokine mediated.

(b) Transcriptase inhibitors increase toxicity.

(c) R human growth factor is of benefit.

(d) Pregabalin is effective.

(e) Topical medication does not help.

14. Phantom limb:

(a) Pain prevalence is influenced by gender.

(b) Congenital amputees have less frequent pain.

(c) Constant pain is a typical feature.

(d) Pain is mostly observed in distal parts of the missing limb.

(e) Phantom pain is more frequent than phantom sensations.

15. Phantom limb:

(a) Phantom sensations fade with time like the phantom.

(b) Flexion of fingers and toes is the most common feeling.

(c) Severe stump pain is seen in 50% of patients.

(d) Increase pain is due to increased and novel expression of sodium channels.

(e) A decrease in grey matter of the thalamus is seen.

16. Phantom limb:

(a) Gabapentin and pregabalin have similar efficacy.

(b) Morphine reduces both stump and phantom pain.

(c) Ketamine infusion decreases phantom pain.

(d) Sympathetic blocks have long-term analgesia benefits.

(e) Spinal cord and deep brain stimulation are beneficial.

17. Alcoholic neuropathy:
    (a) Incidence is almost 50%.
    (b) Paraesthesia is the earliest symptom.
    (c) Mostly is a sensorimotor neuropathy.
    (d) Mostly is a large fibre neuropathy.
    (e) Poor diet contributes to it.

18. Trigeminal neuralgia:
    (a) Has a female preponderance.
    (b) Has a risk factor in multiple sclerosis.
    (c) Most common cause is arterial compression of the trigeminal nerve.
    (d) Pain is continuous.
    (e) Pontine plaques causing damage are seen.

19. Trigeminal neuralgia:
    (a) Pain is precipitated by trigger points.
    (b) Pain is associated with neurological deficits.
    (c) Diagnosis is mainly based on history.
    (d) Mostly bilateral pain is seen.
    (e) Ophthalmic division is most commonly affected.

20. Trigeminal neuralgia:
    (a) Major trigger factor is touching of involved area.
    (b) Anhedonia and depression are common accompaniments.
    (c) Allodynia and sensory loss are seen.
    (d) Diffusion tensor imaging is better than MRI for diagnosis.
    (e) Carbamazepine is beneficial in 100% of patients.

21. Trigeminal neuralgia:
    (a) Carbamazepine causes fluid retention and hyponatremia.
    (b) Incidence of side effects increase with oxcarbamazepine.
    (c) Anaesthesia dolorosa can occur with gasserian ganglion surgery.
    (d) Radio-frequency rhizotomy has long-term benefits.
    (e) Balloon compression rhizolysis has no side effects.

22. Trigeminal neuralgia:
    (a) Glycerol rhizotomy has good long-term benefit.
    (b) Stereotactic radiosurgery can cause facial numbness and paraesthesias.
    (c) Posterior fossa microsurgery is the most effective treatment.

(d) Corneal numbness can occur after posterior fossa microsurgery.
(e) Diplopia is seen secondary to damage to cranial nerves IV and VI and is permanent.

23. Trigeminal neuralgia:
    (a) The presence of trigger zone is pathognomonic.
    (b) May be caused by tumours in cerebellopontine angle.
    (c) Atypical TN responds well to single-agent treatment.
    (d) Tooth extraction can cause trigeminal neuralgia.
    (e) Pain relief is longer with microvascular decompression.

24. Glossopharyngeal neuralgia:
    (a) Most common cause is vascular compression of glossopharyngeal nerve.
    (b) Is mostly unilateral.
    (c) Imaging of choice is MRI.
    (d) Spontaneous remission is seen in 75% of patients.
    (e) Microvascular compression is free of side effects.

25. Complex regional pain syndrome:
    (a) Type 1 is secondary to nerve injury.
    (b) Pain can be triggered with loud noise and emotions.
    (c) Swelling and pain develops at the site of the trauma.
    (d) Type 1 is more common than type 2
    (e) Extremity pain is symmetric in type 1.

26. CRPS
    (a) Pain is more in limbs in dependent position.
    (b) Stimulus-evoked pain is a striking clinical feature.
    (c) No sensory loss is seen.
    (d) Cold CRPS has more favourable course.
    (e) Mechanical hyperalgesia is most commonly seen in warm CRPS.

27. CRPS:
    (a) Hyperhidrosis is more frequent than hypohidrosis.
    (b) Trophic changes are seen early.
    (c) Gross motor movements are affected.
    (d) Tremor may be seen.
    (e) Voluntary movements of limbs are affected less than passive movements.

28. CRPS:
    (a) Upper extremity is more commonly involved.
    (b) Patients show high tendency towards somatisation.
    (c) Increased association is seen with HLA A3, B7 and DR2.
    (d) Vasodilation is seen in denervated area.
    (e) CRPS patients have increased alpha-adrenoceptor density in skin biopsy.

29. CRPS:
    (a) Neurogenic inflammation is seen causing oedema and vasodilation.
    (b) Increased protein concentration is seen in synovial fluid along with synovial hypervascularity.
    (c) TNFα, IL-1 and IL-8 are increased in chronic CRPS patients.
    (d) Dystonia of hands and feet is seen in 50% of patients.
    (e) Budapest score has a sensitivity of 99%.

30. CRPS:
    (a) Bone scintigraphy has high specificity.
    (b) X-ray and bone densitometry are helpful in early stage.
    (c) Post-traumatic neuralgia presents like classic CRPS.
    (d) Intravenous lidocaine has shown efficacy only in type-1 CRPS.
    (e) Epidural clonidine has shown effect in refractory CRPS.

31. CRPS:
    (a) Lower density of C and A fibres are found in affected limbs.
    (b) Lower limb is more affected in paediatric population.
    (c) Substance P and bradykinin contribute to hyperalgesia and allodynia.
    (d) Most common initiating injury is a fracture.
    (e) Main assessment of autonomic function is by thermoregulation and sudomotor regulation.

32. Spinal cord injury
    (a) Most common cause of pain is musculoskeletal pain.
    (b) Below-level neuropathic pain is short-lived.
    (c) Neuropathic pain is more common in people with incomplete lesions.
    (d) Psychological factors are more closely associated with incidence and severity of pain than physical factors.
    (e) Muscle spasm pain is common especially in complete injuries.

33. Spinal cord injury:
    (a) Visceral pain remains accurately localised in tetraplegics.
    (b) Neuropathic pain is mainly on the basis of clinical features.
    (c) At-level neuropathic pain is mostly unilateral.
    (d) Syringomyelia presents with a rising level of sensory loss.
    (e) Cauda equina is a variant of at-level neuropathic pain.

34. Spinal cord injury:
    (a) Below-level neuropathic pain is caudal to the level of spinal cord injury.
    (b) Pain is typically seen below a single dermatome.
    (c) Sudden noise may trigger pain.
    (d) Complete lesions exhibit more allodynia.
    (e) Catastrophising and self-efficacy play an important role in determining disability.

35. Spinal cord injury:
    (a) At-level pain is dependent on preservation of superficial dorsal horn.
    (b) Pain is mediated due to increase in glutaminergic excitatory activity at NMDA, non-NMDA and metabotropic glutamate receptors.
    (c) Microglia are protective against neuropathic pain.
    (d) Reorganisation of cortex is seen in patients with complete thoracic injuries.
    (e) Neuronal loss is seen in thalamus.

36. Spinal cord injury:
    (a) Shoulder pain seen is independent of the level of injury.
    (b) Headache may be a sign of bowel impaction.
    (c) Clonidine intrathecally has shown promise in neuropathic pain.
    (d) Intravenous lignocaine infusion has been associated with good analgesia.
    (e) Intrathecal baclofen is helpful in pinch-induced and musculoskeletal pain.

37. Spinal cord injury:
    (a) TENS is helpful in patients with neuropathic pain below the level of the injury.
    (b) TENS has no side effects.
    (c) Spinal cord stimulation is useful in incomplete lesions.
    (d) Dorsal root entry root lesions have no efficacy.
    (e) Mainstay of shoulder pain is exercises.

38. Spinal cord injury:
    (a) Autonomic dysreflexia accompanies below-level pain.
    (b) Grey matter damage is important for development of below-level pain.
    (c) Elimination of lamina I NK1R expressing neurons can increase spontaneous behaviour.
    (d) Frontal blood flow is increased after spinal cord injury.
    (e) High progesterone states delay onset and attenuates severity of pain.

39. Central pain:
    (a) Main feature is pain/dysesthesias with partial or complete sensory loss.
    (b) Spontaneous pain may be accompanied by allodynia and hyperalgesia.
    (c) Pain is seen in 90% of patients after stroke.
    (d) Musculoskeletal pain is the most common after the stroke.
    (e) High incidence is seen with brainstem infarctions.

40. Central Pain:
    (a) Onset of pain takes at least 6 months.
    (b) No loss of sensory function is seen.
    (c) Abnormal temperature and pain sensibility are most consistent abnormalities.
    (d) Cold allodynia is typically seen in multiple sclerosis.
    (e) Spastic seizures are seen in multiple sclerosis.

41. Multiple sclerosis:
    (a) Acute inflammatory lesions are seen in internal capsule and cerebral peduncle.
    (b) Flexion of the neck may cause electrical sensation.
    (c) Bilateral trigeminal neuralgia may be seen.
    (d) Pain induced by spasms can be triggered by urinary tract infections.
    (e) Pain with flexor spasms is a musculoskeletal pain.

42. Multiple sclerosis:
    (a) Is due to acute inflammation of central myelin.
    (b) Chronic pain is seen in less than 10% of patients.
    (c) Trigeminal sensory loss is more common than normal population.
    (d) Intrathecal baclofen is useful in lower limb extremity.
    (e) Deafferentation pain is a major accompaniment.

43. Syringomyelia:
    (a) Is a cystic cavity in the central canal of the spinal cord.
    (b) Arnold chiari malformation is a frequent accompaniment.
    (c) Is always congenital.
    (d) Pain is abolished as spinothalamic function is lost.
    (e) Spontaneous pain is seen due to deafferentation.

44. Parkinson's disease:
    (a) Manifest as pain in less than 10% of patients.
    (b) Pain is mostly musculoskeletal in late disease.
    (c) Changes in heat pain thresholds are seen as a part of the pain process.
    (d) Basal ganglia are involved in nociceptive process.
    (e) Levodopa is helpful in managing the chronic pain.

45. Central Pain:
    (a) Quantitative sensory testing is helpful in diagnosis.
    (b) Allodynia is more common in patients with normal tactile sensibility.
    (c) Specific pain scales for central pain have been developed.
    (d) Major transmission system involved is spinothalamic system.
    (e) Allodynia/dysesthesia is more frequent in patients with pain.

46. Central pain:
    (a) Burning pain seen is because of thalamic involvement.
    (b) Stimulation of anterior cingulate ameliorates the pain.
    (c) Increase in cerebral blood flow is seen in spontaneous central pain.
    (d) Increased release of excitatory amino acids can cause sensitisation and hypertrophy in syringomyelia.
    (e) Abnormalities of sodium channels may contribute to pain in syringomyelia.

47. Central pain:
    (a) Amitriptyline is useful in mixed type of pain.
    (b) Duloxetine is helpful in allodynia.
    (c) Pregabalin is drug of choice in pain with anxiety and spasticity.
    (d) Dronabinol has no efficacy in central pain.
    (e) Transcranial magnetic stimulation is effective.

48. Central pain:
    (a) Is always unilateral
    (b) Can manifest as diabetic neuropathy.
    (c) Most common pain is burning type.
    (d) Most patients with allodynia get relief on movements of the limbs.
    (e) Ataxia is seen more than hemiplegia.

✅ Answers

1. T F T F T
   Varicella causes chicken pox during the first contact and stays dormant by body's cell-mediated immunity. It is associated with decrease in cell-mediated immunity and is seen in >85% of patients more than 85 years of age. Risk factors include increased age, severity of rash during the acute phase and greater acute pain severity. Female to male ratio is 3:2. Most common sites are ophthalmic (32%), thoracic (16.5%) and facial (16%).

2. T F T T T
   Virus moves along affected sensory nerves and produces unilateral rash. Inflammatory changes seen are loss of cells, myelin, axons with ganglionic fibrosis and atrophy of dorsal horn.

3. F T F F T
   Maculopapular vesicular rash is seen causing burning sensation. In acute phase, antiretroviral medications (acyclovir, valaciclovir, famciclovir) are effective if started within 72 hours. Topical lidocaine has NNT of 2.0, anti-convulsants (4.3–4.9) and opioids (4.6).

4. T F F T F
   Doses less than 200 mg/day of venlafaxine only inhibit serotonin reup-take and do not have any analgesic effect, whereas doses greater than 200 mg/day inhibits norepinephrine reuptake which is essential for anal-gesia. Opioids are effective in high doses. Intrathecal methylprednisolone is effective though there is risk of adhesive arachnoiditis.

5. F F T T T
   The neuropathies seen are acute sensory neuropathy, chronic sensorimotor distal neuropathy and autonomic neuropathy. The risk factors are age and duration of diabetes, impaired glucose tolerance, obesity with decreased LDL and increased plasma triglycerides.

6. F T T F T

Sorbitol and fructose concentrations are seen in nerves leading to decrease in Na-K ATPase activity. Nitric oxide and glutathione concentrations are decreased which acts as buffer against oxidative injury and vasodilation causing chronic ischaemia. Neuronal ischaemia is seen because of thickening of capillary basement membrane along with endothelial cell hyperplasia. Chronic hyperglycaemia leads to deposition of advanced glycosylation products around peripheral nerves. NADPH increases hydrogen peroxide and increases oxidative stress.

7. T F F F T

Sensorimotor neuropathy is seen in more than 80% of patients. Most commonly feet are involved. Mostly small fibres are involved. Loss of touch and pain is seen before pressure and vibration because of involvement of large-diameter fibres.

8. T F T T F

The differential diagnosis includes peripheral vascular disease, restless legs syndrome, vitamin B12 deficiency, hypothyroidism and uraemia. Autonomic neuropathy is seen in both type 1 and type 2 diabetes. Neuropathy can cause loss of sympathetic tone and vasodilation causing pooling of blood in lower extremities. Diabetic amyotrophy is only seen in type 2 and is characterised by pain and weakness along with atrophy of proximal lower limb muscles.

9. F F F F T

Mononeuropathies mainly involve ulnar and median nerve. Most effective treatment is tight glycaemic control and which is more effective in patients without retinopathy. Gabapentin has a NNT of four for 50% reduction in pain.

10. T F F T F

Mononeuropathies are commonly seen especially of motor nerves of extracellular muscles. Most common nerve palsy is third nerve palsy and is due to involvement of nervi nervorum. Arteriolar changes are seen without vascular occlusion. Diabetic amyotrophy is predominantly asymmetric motor neuropathy which is painful.

11. T F T T T
Polyneuropathy is most commonly seen. Neuropathy is seen in 10–35% of patients. Sensory neuropathy seen is distal sensory neuropathy. The risk factors include older age, advanced disease state, nutritional deficit, use of dideoxynucleoside reverse transcriptase inhibitors and exposure to protease and alcohol.

12. T T F T F
Soles are involved first with progression up. Numbness is the initial symptom followed by burning sensation. Loss of ankle reflex may be seen.

13. T T T T F
HIV-related neuropathy is not virus mediated as virus does not affect axons or Schwann cells.

14. F T F T F
Phantom limb is not influenced by age in adults, gender, side/level of amputation and cause of amputation. Pain is present on an intermittent basis (daily or weekly).

15. F T F T T
Phantom fades with time and not the sensations (shrinkage or telescoping). Severe stump pain is seen in 5–10% of patients. Increased sodium channels are also seen in dorsal root ganglion.

16. F T T F T
Only gabapentin has shown efficacy.

17. F T T F T

18. T T T F T
Trigeminal neuralgia is seen more in females. The risk factors include multiple sclerosis, (where it is seen bilaterally as opposed to more common unilateral form), increased age and hypertension. The trigeminal nerve is compressed in the root entry zone, which is an area of transition from central to peripheral myelin which is sensitive to pressure. The pain is in paroxysms and is because of demyelination and extra-synaptic transmission of impulses.

19. T F T F F
Only 4% manifest as bilateral pain, while 60% have right-sided predominance. Most commonly involved are mandibular and maxillary.

20. F T T T F
Major precipitating factor is chewing and talking (76%) followed by
touching (65%) and cold (48%). Allodynia and sensory loss are seen especially in atypical trigeminal neuralgia. Demyelination is associated with
changes in water diffusion that can be detected by diffusion tracer imag-
ing. Carbamazepine is beneficial in 70% of patients.

21. T F T T F
Carbamazepine causes fluid retention and hyponatremia along with osteoporosis, neutropenia and megaloblastic anaemia. Oxcarbamazepine is
excreted renally, so it has less side effects. Gasserian ganglion is approached
through the foramen ovale and may cause numbness, increased recurrence,
cardiac arrhythmias, cardiac arrest and anaesthesia dolorosa (severe constant pain associated with numbness). Radio frequency has recurrence rate
of 40% at 5 years. Balloon compression causes ischaemic damage to rootlets
and ganglion cells. Side effects include transient masseter weakness, vascular injury and aseptic meningitis.

22. F T T T F
The recurrence is seen within 3 years of glycerol rhizotomy. Posterior
fossa microsurgery is the most effective treatment with 73% having complete pain relief at 5 years. It is associated with corneal numbness, meningitis, cerebral infarcts, GI bleeding, pulmonary emboli and diplopia.
Diplopia seen is transient.

23. T T F T T
Trigger points are less than 10 mm in the oral mucosa or perineal area.
Atypical TN is usually resistant to single agent and surgery. Extraction of
the third molar is especially associated with TN.

24. T T T T F
Microvascular compression is associated with dysphoria, dysphagia,
hypoacusis and CSF leak.

25. F T F T F
Type 1 is secondary to trauma whereas type 2 is secondary to major
nerve injury. Swelling and pain develops remote to the site of the injury.

Type 1 is more common than type 2 in arms than legs. Also it is more in females as compared to males. The peak age seen is around 37–50 years. Extremity pain is asymmetric without an overt nerve lesion.

26. T T F F T
   In CRPS 1, initially the affected limb is warm than the contralateral limb. Initial decrease in temperature has an unfavourable prognosis.

27. T F F T F
   Abnormal nail growth, decreased or increased hair growth, fibrosis, thin glossy skin and osteoporosis are late changes and seen in chronic patients. Small accurate movements are affected. Tremor seen is extension of physiological tremor.

28. T T T T T
   Upper extremity is more commonly involved with a preponderance for left side. Vasodilation is seen in denervated area with increased sensitivity to catecholamines seen in later stages.

29. T T F F T
   The markers are only increased in acute phase. Dystonia of hands and feet is seen only in 10% of patients.

30. T F F F T
   Bone scintigraphy has specificity of 75–100% and sensitivity of 31–69%. Pathological uptake in the metacarpophalangeal or metacarpal bones is thought to be sensitive and specific. X-ray and bone densitometry are helpful in early stage and show endosteal and intracortical extravasation, subperiosteal and trabecular bone resorption, spotty and localised demineralisation and osteoporosis. Post-traumatic neuralgia presents with spontaneous burning pain, and associated hyperalgesia and cold allodynia are confined to the territory of the nerve. Intravenous lidocaine is effective in both type 1 and type 2. High dosage of epidural clonidine (700 mg) is more effective than lower dosage (300 mg).

31. T T T T T
   Lower limb is affected up to 5 times more in paediatric population and is mostly seen after puberty. Females are predominantly involved in paediatric population. Thermoregulation is measured by thermoregulation sweat test, while sudomotor regulation is measured by quantitative sudomotor axon reflex test.

32. T F T T F

Musculoskeletal pain is seen above the level of the lesion (58%), at-level pain is seen in 42% of patients and below-level pain is seen in 34% of patients. Severe or excruciating neuropathic pain develops months to years following injury. Psychological factors like disturbed mood and acceptance of disability can affect severity of pain. Muscle spasms are more common in incomplete lesions.

33. F T T T T

Visceral pain presents as vague unpleasantness which is difficult to interpret. Syringomyelia is a cyst or cavity formation in the spinal cord. It presents as delayed onset of segmental pain and is mostly seen 5–6 years after the injury. Cauda equina seen is due to nerve root damage. Pain is reported in lower lumbar and sacral dermatomes and is mostly a burning, stabbing hot type.

34. T F T F T

Below-level lesion is seen at least three dermatomes below the lesion. Incomplete lesions are more likely to exhibit allodynia because of sparing of tracts conveying touch sensation.

35. T T F T T

Ablation of structures in superficial dorsal horn can relieve at-level pain. Microglia are instrumental in developing below-level neuropathic pain.

36. T T T T F

Headache in upper thoracic or cervical spinal cord injury may be because of visceral disturbance like bowel impaction or bladder distension causing autonomic dysreflexia. Though intravenous lignocaine is helpful, oral congeners (mexiletine) have not shown much evidence for the pain management. Intrathecal baclofen is helpful in neuropathic and muscle spasm pain.

37. F F T F T

TENS is helpful more in pain at the level of the injury. TENS may cause detrusor sphincter dyssynergia. Dorsal root entry root lesioning is useful in unilateral, radicular cauda equina pain. Those with sacral, continuous pain, below-level neuropathic pain or a syrinx are less likely to do well.

38. T T F T T
    Autonomic dysreflexia is a potential life-threatening condition causing increase or decrease of blood pressure and pulse, headache, cerebral haemorrhage, CVS collapse and seizures. Elimination of lamina I NK1R-expressing neurons decreases injury-induced at-level spontaneous pain behaviour.

39. T T F T T
    Central pain is the pain caused by a lesion or disease of the central somatosensory nervous system. Dysesthesia is the presence of unpleasant sensations along with pain. Hyperalgesia is increased pain response to a stimulus that normally produces pain. Pain is seen in 1–50% of patients after stroke. Musculoskeletal pain is most common (40%) followed by shoulder pain (20%), headache (10%), central pain (10%) and spasticity (7%). Central pain is mostly seen with lateral medullary infarction and those involving the inferolateral part of thalamus.

40. F F T T F
    Onset of central pain is seen within a month in two-thirds of patients. Ninety percent of patients show loss of cold, warmth and pinprick sensation. Pain is mostly in the form of tonic seizures which are paroxysms of painful attacks lasting couple of minutes with pain on the face and arm. The leg is associated with abnormal or dystonic postures.

41. T T T T T
    Lhermitte's sign is a sudden and short-lasting electric sensation spreading down the spine from the cervical region on flexion of the neck. Pain induced by spasms can be triggered by urinary infection along with tactile stimulation, full bladder and emotional factors. Flexor spasms are seen due to repeated muscular contractions.

42. T F T T T

43. T T F T T
    If the cavity extends into the brainstem, it is called as syringobulbia. Noncongenital cases of syringomyelia are mostly seen with spinal cord injury. Pain is seen even after the abolition of the spinothalamic tract.

44. F F T T T

There are 40–75% of patients present with pain. Pain is musculoskeletal in the early disease, and with progression it becomes musculoskeletal, nociceptive and neuropathic.

45. T T F T T

QST is helpful for documenting sensory loss and the presence of hypersensitivity. No specific scale exists, and the most commonly used scales are visual analogue scale and numerical rating scale.

46. T F F T T

Disruption of thermosensory integration leads to disinhibition of noxious responding thalamocortical neurons causing burning pain. Spontaneous central pain is associated with decrease in regional cerebral blood flow in the thalamus contralateral to the side of the pain. Alterations in Nav1.3 channels are seen in syringomyelia.

47. F T F F T

Amitriptyline is not effective in mixed pain (nociceptive and neuropathic) in spinal cord injury. It is also more useful in patients with pain associated with depression. Duloxetine is helpful in dynamic mechanical and cold allodynia. Pregabalin is the drug of choice for pain and anxiety because of its anxiolytic effect. Gabapentin has some antispasmodic effect and hence useful in spasticity. Dronabinol is an orally administered synthetic Δ9-tetrahydrocannabinol which is effective with a low NNT of 3.4–3.7.

48. T T T F T

Central pain can present as diabetic neuropathy but is peripheral with damage to Aδ and C fibres. It is mostly seen as bilateral. Most common type of pain is burning pain (40–60%), followed by aching (30–40%), lancinating (7–30%) and pricking (6–30%). Movement of limbs causes increase in pain in 70% of patients while relief in 20% of patients. Ataxia is seen in 60% of patients, while hemiplegia is seen in 35% of patients.

Deep Somatic Tissue Pain

© Springer International Publishing AG 2018
R. Gupta, *Multiple Choice Questions in Pain Management*,
DOI 10.1007/978-3-319-56917-8_6

❓ Questions

1. Joint pain:
   (a) Pain is elicited by stimulation of normal cartilage and synovial tissue.
   (b) Most common presentation is persistent pain at rest.
   (c) Is mainly mediated by Aβ fibres.
   (d) Cartilage is richly innervated with Aδ fibres.
   (e) Vast majority of articular sensory neurons are isolectin B4+ve.

2. Joint pain:
   (a) Chronic persistent hyperalgesia is because of increased mechanosensitivity.
   (b) Mechano-insensitive silent nociceptors comprise mainly of C fibres.
   (c) PGI2 released has a fast onset than PGE2.
   (d) Substance P increases mechanosensitivity in afferents.
   (e) Increased C-fos expression is seen in lamina I.

3. Joint pain:
   (a) NMDA receptors are activated on non-noxious stimuli.
   (b) Increased glutamate is seen in acute inflammation.
   (c) Joint inflammation leads to decrease in spinal COX-2.
   (d) Arthroplasty reverses pain-induced changes in the central nervous system.
   (e) Intrathecal administration of A1 adenosine agonists inhibits inflammation and joint destruction.

4. Muscle pain:
   (a) Is seen in 90% of population.
   (b) Is associated with autonomic phenomenon.
   (c) Muscle nociceptors are free nerve endings.
   (d) Free nerve ending exons are thickly myelinated.
   (e) Muscle nociceptors are usually high-threshold mechanosensitive receptors.

5. Muscle pain:
   (a) ATP causes pain by binding to purinergic membrane receptors (P2X3).
   (b) Vanilloid receptor TRPV1 elicits pain in muscle.
   (c) Nerve growth factor inhibition is seen in inflamed muscle.
   (d) Nociceptive input from muscle is processed in lamina IV–VI.
   (e) Nerve growth factor causes long-standing allodynia.

6. Arthritis:
   (a) Osteoarthritis is the most common form.
   (b) Pain with use of joint is typical in osteoarthritis.
   (c) Radiographic changes are seen early in osteoarthritis.
   (d) Osteoarthritis is seen more commonly in females.
   (e) Density of the bone is increased in osteoarthritis.

7. Osteoarthritis:
   (a) Has a strong heritable component.
   (b) Low serum levels of vitamin C increases the risk of knee OA.
   (c) Selenium deficiency is involved with endemic form of arthritis.
   (d) Acetabular dysplasia increases the incidence of hip osteoarthritis.
   (e) Premature apoptosis and senescence are characteristics of osteoarthritis chondrocytes.

8. Osteoarthritis:
   (a) Bones show increased thickness and volume.
   (b) Pain is primarily due to the stretch of the cartilage.
   (c) Temporomandibular pain may be an accompaniment.
   (d) Topical capsaicin is useful.
   (e) Surgery has better outcome for knee OA than hip OA.

9. Osteoarthritis:
   (a) Atrophic form is associated with younger population.
   (b) Affects any synovial joint of the body.
   (c) Most common deformity is valgus deformity.
   (d) Hand OA has predilection for females.
   (e) Pain may come from the bone marrow.

10. Osteoarthritis:
    (a) Synovial hypertrophy is seen more than the effusions.
    (b) May present with crystals in tissues and synovial fluids.
    (c) Capsaicin cream can cause burning and rash.
    (d) Intraarticular steroids are most helpful in knee osteoarthritis.
    (e) Obesity prevention can help reduce incidence.

11. Rheumatoid arthritis:
    (a) Involves peripheral synovial joints.
    (b) Joint involvement is symmetrical.
    (c) Morning stiffness is short-lived.

    (d) Extraarticular organ involvement is seen.
    (e) Rheumatoid factor is detected in 40% of patients.

12. Rheumatoid arthritis:
    (a) Positive rheumatoid factor is specific for rheumatoid arthritis.
    (b) ACPA is highly sensitive for rheumatoid arthritis.
    (c) Heritability is seen up to the extent of 90%.
    (d) Cigarette smoke is a risk factor.
    (e) Synovium is only infiltrated by macrophages.

13. Rheumatoid arthritis:
    (a) Molecular signals lead to synovial hypertrophy.
    (b) Synovial hypertrophy is due to hypoxia.
    (c) Agents that inhibit or slow bone resorption suppress inflammation.
    (d) Disease-modifying drugs are started early in the disease.
    (e) TNF inhibitory treatment is associated with reactivation of latent tuberculosis.

14. Rheumatoid arthritis:
    (a) Neutropenia may be seen.
    (b) Metacarpal changes are earliest on the X-rays.
    (c) Radial drift of metacarpophalangeal joints is characteristic.
    (d) Gold salts can cause skin and blood dyscrasias.
    (e) Patients are at risk for C3–C4 subluxation.

15. Systemic lupus erythematosus:
    (a) Has a predilection for males.
    (b) May present as fever.
    (c) Major symptom is photosensitivity.
    (d) ANA is positive in 98% of patients.
    (e) Pregnancy can cause flaring of symptoms.

16. Temporal arteritis:
    (a) Is seen more commonly in female than males.
    (b) Infiltration of lymphocytes and the presence of giant cells are diagnostic.
    (c) Has a predilection for venous system.
    (d) Sudden onset of blindness may be seen.
    (e) Temporal artery biopsy is diagnostic.

17. Polymyalgia rheumatica:
    (a) Most commonly pelvic muscles are involved.
    (b) Has a better response to treatment than frozen shoulder.
    (c) Malignancy may present as PMR.
    (d) Drug of choice is oral steroids.
    (e) Is a disease of young population.

18. Fibromyalgia:
    (a) Eleven of 18 tender points must exhibit painful sensitivity to 4 kg of digital palpation pressure.
    (b) Palpation of tender points may lead to lacrimation.
    (c) Is mostly seen in males.
    (d) Insomnia is a major accompaniment.
    (e) Naproxen can help in treatment of headaches caused by caffeine withdrawal.

19. Fibromyalgia:
    (a) Most common headache seen is migraine.
    (b) Most effective treatment is analgesics.
    (c) Morning stiffness has more duration in fibromyalgia than in rheumatoid arthritis.
    (d) Fatigue is rarely seen.
    (e) Bipolar disorder is commonly seen.

20. Fibromyalgia:
    (a) Most common gastrointestinal conditions involved are inflammatory bowel syndrome and benign dyspepsia.
    (b) Urinary symptoms are more frequent in males.
    (c) Skeletal muscle degeneration is seen.
    (d) Lack of endogenous opioids is a cause for central pain.
    (e) Exercise improves symptoms in fibromyalgia.

21. Fibromyalgia:
    (a) Fatigue is mostly disabling and worse in the morning.
    (b) Poor sleep is seen in 20% of patients.
    (c) Anxiety is prominent component.
    (d) Stiffness is short-lived.
    (e) Unexplained weight loss and fever are common.

22. Fibromyalgia:
    (a) Symptom severity scale is based on fatigue, waking unrefreshed and cognitive symptoms.
    (b) Joint swelling and muscle weakness may be seen.
    (c) Familial major mood disorder is a risk factor.
    (d) Secondary hyperalgesia is increased in fibromyalgia.
    (e) Levels of substance P, serotonin and nerve growth factor are increased in cerebrospinal fluid.

23. Fibromyalgia:
    (a) Sleep deprivation can lead to sensitisation and myalgia.
    (b) Reduced hypothalamic-pituitary-adrenal axis response is seen.
    (c) Exercise increases pain and should be avoided.
    (d) Duloxetine has shown efficacy.
    (e) Low titres of autoantibodies may be seen.

24. Postmastectomy pain:
    (a) Is seen in 10% of patients after breast surgery.
    (b) Most common cause is bone pain.
    (c) Phantom pain can be seen.
    (d) Increased body weight is a risk factor.
    (e) TENS can decrease the incidence of neurosis and pain after mastectomy.

25. Post-thoracotomy pain:

    (a) Pain seen after 3 months of surgical procedure.
    (b) Injury of the intercostal nerves is the main cause.
    (c) Pleurectomy is protective.
    (d) Incidence is 20% after thoracotomy.
    (e) Radio-frequency ablation of dorsal root ganglion is a more effective treatment than pulsed radio frequency.

✔️ Answers

1. F T F F F
   Pain is mostly poorly localised and dull. Pain is mostly mediated by C fibres (80%) followed by Aβ and Aδ fibres. Cartilage is not innervated by any nerve fibres. Aδ and C fibres terminate as free nerve endings in fibrous capsule, adipose tissue, ligaments, menisci, periosteum and synovial layer. Sensory neurons are mostly peptidergic and isolectin B4−ve.

2. T F T T T
Mechano-insensitive silent nociceptors are comprised of one-third of
C fibres and Aδ fibres. Substance P and vasoactive intestinal peptide
increase mechanosensitivity, while endomorphin 1 and somatostatin
decrease the same.

3. F T F T T
NMDA receptors are activated on noxious stimuli. Glutamate receptors
play an important role in generation and maintenance of inflammation-
evoked spinal hyperexcitability. Joint inflammation leads to increase in
spinal COX-2 and increased release of PGE2 in dorsal and ventral horn.
Arthroplasty reverses the atrophy of the thalamus and grey matter of the
cerebrum seen with chronic joint pain.

4. F T T F T
Autonomic phenomena seen are hypotension and sweating. Muscle nociceptors are beadlike structures connected by thin stretches of axons. Free
nerve endings are thinly myelinated (gp III with a velocity of 2.5–30 cm/s)
or nonmyelinated (gp IV with a velocity of 0.4–2.5 cm/s). Forty percent of
muscle nociceptors are low-threshold mechanosensitive receptors which
work as ergoreceptors (helps and adjusts respiration and circulation during the exercise).

5. T T F T T
ATP is released from damaged muscle cells. TRPV1 receptor is proton
sensitive, and intramuscular injection causes pain. Nerve growth factor is
a neurotrophic factor and neuropeptide involved in the survival of neurons. Nerve growth factor synthesis is increased in inflamed muscle.

6. T T F T T
Osteoarthritis is typically seen in lower extremities. Radiological changes
are seen late in disease and include joint space narrowing, osteophytes,
sclerosis and cysts. MRI may show cartilage loss, osteophytes, bone marrow
lesions, synovitis and effusions. Osteoarthritis is seen in 47% of females as
compared to 40% of males. Density of the bone is increased though the
bone is less mineralised.

7. F T T T T
Osteoarthritis has a strong heritable component for hand and hip disease. Kashin-Beck osteoarthropathy in China is associated with selenium
and iodine deficiency.

8. T F T T F
   Bone in OA has a high turnover state causing hypomineralisation and weak bone. Cartilage is aneural. The pain is felt due to medullary hypertension and microfractures along with inflammation of the synovium. COMT polymorphism contributes to low back, neck and TMJ pain. Topical capsaicin releases substance P and CGRP and depletes nociceptors of transmitter peptides. Surgery has better outcome for hip osteoarthritis (almost 100%) than knee OA (30%).

9. T T F T T
   Atrophic form is seen in younger population and is characterised by synovial inflammation and bone erosion, whereas hypertrophic form is seen in older population and is characterised by overgrowth of bones around affected joints. The disease mainly affects apophyseal joints of spine (mid-cervical and lumbar), interphalangeal, carpometacarpal joints, knee and hip. The ankle is least likely to be affected. Medial tibiofemoral joint involvement leads to varus deformity. Hand involvement leads to swelling of distal (Heberden's nodes) and proximal (Bouchard's) joints. The periosteum, subchondral and bone marrow can cause pain. Increased intraosseous pressure arising from impaired venous drainage causes pain.

10. F T T T T
    Effusions are seen in 34% of patients while synovial hypertrophy is seen in 17% of patients. Calcium pyrophosphate dihydrate (CPPD) is a marker of hypertrophic form, whereas basic calcium phosphate (BCP) is a marker of atrophic form.

11. T T F T F
    Rheumatoid arthritis is an immune-mediated, chronic inflammatory polyarthritis. Unlike osteoarthritis where stiffness is short-lived, rheumatoid arthritis has stiffness lasting greater than 2 h. Extraarticular involvement is seen in the form of rheumatoid nodules especially on elbows, pleural disease, scleritis, xerostomia, Baker's cyst (effusions in the knees) and erosion of odontoid process. Rheumatoid factor is an autoantibody against Fc portion of IgG and is detectable in 85% of patients. RF titres >1:160 dilution are highly suggestive of the disease. High titres signify severe disease.

12. F T F T F
    Rheumatoid factor can present with other chronic inflammatory infectious conditions. High levels of rheumatoid factor in disease are associ-

ated with poor prognosis. Anticyclic citrullinated peptide antibodies (ACPA) are directed against citrullinated residues of peptides and with higher specificity (95%) and sensitivity (70%). There is 50–60% association with HLA-DR4 risk factors including cigarette smoke, female gender (2.5:1) and bacterial and viral agents. Synovium is infiltrated by macrophages, fibroblasts, leucocytes, dendritic cells, B cells, T cells, mast cells and NK cells.

13. T T F T T

Pannus or proliferative synovial tissue is due to hypoxia of synovium because of increased metabolic demands. Agents that inhibit or slow bone resorption do not suppress inflammation. Bone erosions are mainly caused by osteoclasts accumulating at the pannus-bone interface. Receptor activator of NF-κB (RANK) along with its ligand RANKL modulates bone resorption. Disease-modifying drugs like methotrexate and leflunomide are started early in the disease.

14. T T F T F

Felty's syndrome comprises of neutropenia, splenomegaly and rheumatoid arthritis. Earliest change on X-ray is seen in second and third metacarpophalangeal joints and third proximal interphalangeal joints. Ulnar drift of metacarpophalangeal joints is characteristic. Patients are at risk for C1–C2 subluxation.

15. F T T T T

SLE may present as acute febrile illness with arthralgia and rash. Forty-four percent of patients show photosensitivity. Pregnancy can cause flaring of symptoms and leads to spontaneous abortions and late-term foetal demise.

16. T T F T T

SLE has a predilection for arteries especially elastin-containing arteries. Twenty percent of patients may have sudden blindness because of ischaemic optic neuritis.

17. F T T T F

Most commonly shoulder and neck pain is seen. Symptoms are mostly bilateral. Response to treatment is rapid with oral steroids as compared to frozen shoulder which is gradual. It is most commonly seen in the elderly (>50 years).

18. T T F T T

Amount of pressure applied can be gauged by pressing the thumb against an unyielding surface until blood in the thumbnail is blanched from its tip to midportion. Nine sites should be bilateral including occiput, low cervical, supraspinatus, trapezius, second rib, lateral epicondyle, gluteal, greater trochanter and medial knee. Palpation of tender points can lead to withdrawal, diffuse activation of the arrector pili of the skin (cutis anserina) and spontaneous lacrimation. The incidence is more in females (3–7 times) than males with a peak seen in the mid-1970s. The variant form seen in childhood does not have a gender preference. Ninety percent of patients may also exhibit obstructive sleep apnoea, and periodic involuntary naproxen can help with the headache but will not eliminate the subsequent desire to resume caffeine use.

19. F F T F T

The most common headache seen is tension-type headache. Most effective treatment for headache in fibromyalgia is a long hot bath or shower with sleep for at least 30 min. Morning stiffness seen in fibromyalgia lasts for 45 min to 4 h as against 30 min in rheumatoid arthritis and 5–15 min in osteoarthritis. Fatigue is seen in 80% of patients.

20. T F F F T

Female urethral syndrome is seen which presents as urinary frequency, dysuria, suprapubic discomfort and urethral pain. Skeletal muscle degeneration is not seen though microscopic changes in the form of mitochondrial abnormalities, atrophy of type 2 muscle fibres and ragged red fibres are seen. Dynorphin A levels in cerebrospinal fluid are either normal or increased. Aerobic exercise increases serotonin levels and may improve symptoms in fibromyalgia.

21. T F T F F

Sixty-five percent of patients have sleep disturbances. Insomnia or difficulty in falling asleep is less common. The sleep disturbance is accompanied by restless leg syndrome in 20–40% of patients. Anxiety seen is associated with dizziness, excess sweating, shortness of breath, dysphagia and palpitations. The stiffness seen lasts the whole day. Weight loss and fever are not seen and suggest alternative diagnosis.

22. T F T T F

They are scored between 0 and 3. A diagnosis is made with widespread pain index (WPI) > 7 and SSS > 5 or WPI > 3–6 and SSS > 9. The presence of joint swelling, muscle weakness, abnormal gait, delayed tendon reflexes and focal neurological signs suggests alternate diagnosis. Other risk factors include somatisation, mental disorder, psychological distress, major depression and panic disorder. Secondary hyperalgesia is pain elicited from tissues around the site of pain. Levels of serotonin are decreased, while that of substance P and nerve growth factor are increased.

23. T T F T T

Sleep deprivation of non-REM sleep can induce symptoms and hyperalgesic tender sites of fibromyalgia. HPA axis dysfunction can manifest as low free cortisol levels in 24 h urine collection, loss of circadian rhythm secretion of cortisol, insulin-induced hypoglycaemia and decreased growth hormone. Exercise increases pain, but physical function, quality of life, sleep and fatigue are improved. Duloxetine is a combined serotonin and norepinephrine reuptake inhibitor and is effective at the dose of 60 mg bd.

24. F F T T T

Pain is seen in 47% of patients after lumpectomy, mastectomy, sentinel or complete lymph node dissection. Most common cause of pain is involvement of intercostobrachial nerve which is a cutaneous sensory branch of T1, T2 and T3. Risk factors include increased body weight, young patients, increased height, prosthesis insertion, postoperative radiotherapy and complete lymph node dissection.

25. F T F F T

Pain is seen after 2 months. Pleurectomy is a strong risk factor for the pain. The pain is seen in 50% of patients.

Visceral Pain

❓ Questions

1. Visceral pain:
   (a) Actual cutting of the intestine may not be perceived as painful.
   (b) Mostly felt at source rather than being referred.
   (c) All visceral afferent fibres terminate in the spinal cord.
   (d) Most afferents are thinly myelinated Aδ fibres and unmyelinated C fibres.
   (e) Referred pain is because of convergence.

2. Visceral pain:
   (a) Visceral neurons contain more substance P and CGRP.
   (b) Visceral DRG shows high reactivity for TRPV1.
   (c) Visceral afferents terminate in lamina I.
   (d) Bilateral transection of spinothalamic tract can abolish the behavioural response to noxious visceral stimuli.
   (e) Posterior insula is the main structure activated on visceral stimulation.

3. Visceral pain:
   (a) Most mechanosensitive afferent fibres respond at high distending pressures.
   (b) Mechanically insensitive afferent fibres (silent nociceptors) are not seen in viscera.
   (c) Ischaemic-sensitive cardiac afferent fibres are triggered by protons and ATP.
   (d) Deletion of Na.v.1.8 leads to decreased visceral sensitivity.
   (e) Only serotonergic ligand-gated channels play an important role in visceral sensation.

4. Visceral pain:
   (a) TRPV1 is decreased in bladder injuries.
   (b) Only TRPV1 contributes to colonic hypersensitivity.
   (c) Pancreatitis-related pain can be reversed by blocking TRPV1 and TRPA1 receptors.
   (d) Cross sensitisation is responsible for multiple organ involvement in visceral pain.
   (e) Functional visceral disorders are not associated with involvement of local mediators.

5. Visceral pain:
   (a) Most visceral sensory neurons are unimodal.
   (b) Serotonin is the main transmitter.
   (c) More strong emotional response is seen to visceral pain than to non-visceral pain.
   (d) Serotonin reuptake inhibitors are helpful in visceral pain.
   (e) Pregabalin has shown efficacy in chronic pancreatitis.

6. Visceral pain:
   (a) Has poor and unreliable localisation.
   (b) True visceral pain is referred to nonvisceral pain.
   (c) Secondary somatic hyperalgesia is seen.
   (d) Abdominal pain is mostly seen in elderly and females.
   (e) Proctalgia fugax is common than levator ani syndrome.

7. Visceral pain:
   (a) Viscera are innervated by one set of primary afferent fibres like non-visceral tissue.
   (b) Visceral afferents have no end organs.
   (c) Spinal afferents are mainly myelinated Aδ and unmyelinated C fibres.
   (d) Visceral afferents terminate in spinal cord laminae I, II, V and X.
   (e) Unilateral anterolateral cordotomy is most useful for diffuse intractable visceral pain.

8. Thoracic pain:
   (a) Sensation of angina can be evoked by thalamic stimulation.
   (b) Mechanical stimuli are more effective than chemical stimuli in pericarditis.
   (c) Suprascapular nerve block effectively abolishes shoulder pain after thoracotomy.
   (d) Dyspnoea is associated with activation of anterior cingulate cortex and insular cortex.
   (e) Main receptor involved in human breast pain is TRPV1.

9. Thoracic pain:
   (a) Pneumonia is associated with pleuritic pain always.
   (b) Most common cause of noncardiac chest pain is GERD.
   (c) Costochondritis is chest pain with localised swelling.
   (d) Major cause of thoracic outlet syndrome is venous occlusion.
   (e) Cyclic mastodynia is relieved with menses.

10. Thoracic pain:
    (a) Non-cyclic mastodynia is mostly bilateral.
    (b) Mastodynia increases the expression of TRPV4 and TRPV3.
    (c) Post-CABG pain can present as hypoesthesia.
    (d) Breast implants lead to decrease in thoracic pain.
    (e) Female gender predisposes to long-term post-thoracotomy pain.

11. Abdominal pain:
    (a) Irritable bowel syndrome is the most common disorder.
    (b) Improvement of pain with vomiting is characteristic in inflammatory bowel syndrome (IBS).
    (c) IBS is more common in males.
    (d) Most common psychiatric association is anxiety disorder.
    (e) Extraintestinal manifestations are more common in males.

12. Inflammatory bowel syndrome:
    (a) Higher-amplitude propagating contractions are responsible for urgency and diarrhoea.
    (b) Patients with ulcerative colitis in remission present with symptoms of IBD.
    (c) Infectious causes account for 70% of cases.
    (d) Rectal threshold for distension is increased.
    (e) Activation of gut-associated immune cells in the intestinal mucosa is one of the inciting mechanisms.

13. Irritable bowel syndrome:
    (a) Enhanced colonic mechano-stimulation is hallmark.
    (b) Hypersensitivity of lumbar splanchnic afferents induces hyperalgesia.
    (c) Pain induced from the upper gut is because of the vagus nerve.
    (d) Expression of TRPV1 in increased in IBD.
    (e) P2X3 receptors are increased in IBD.

14. Irritable bowel syndrome:
    (a) High-altitude propagated contractions are decreased.
    (b) Enhanced perception of visceral stimuli is seen.
    (c) Higher pressures are needed in intestine and rectosigmoid to cause pain.
    (d) Has hypersensitivity to rectal stimulation as like functional dyspepsia.
    (e) Increased activation of dorsal anterior cingulate cortex.

15. Irritable bowel syndrome:
    (a) Association with fibromyalgia shows greater activation of dorsal ACC subregion.
    (b) Mucosal inflammation is seen.
    (c) Mast cell is the main component in mucosa of patients.
    (d) Decreased immunoreactivity for TRPV1 is seen.
    (e) Increased IL-1 levels are seen.

16. Irritable bowel syndrome:
    (a) Is seen in 40% of the population.
    (b) Constipation is the most common presentation.
    (c) Males are affected more than the females.
    (d) Association is seen with anxiety disorders.
    (e) Is associated with bacterial overgrowth.

17. Irritable bowel syndrome:
    (a) Dietary control helps alleviate symptoms.
    (b) 5HT3 antagonists are helpful in the treatment.
    (c) Faecal incontinence is a matter of severity.
    (d) 5HT4 antagonists are not helpful in treating symptoms.
    (e) Hypnotherapy helps control the symptoms.

18. Functional dyspepsia:
    (a) Is a diagnosis of exclusion.
    (b) Post-prandial fullness is one of the diagnostic criteria.
    (c) Symptoms get worse with time.
    (d) Delayed gastric emptying is seen.
    (e) *H. pylori* eradication leads to improvement in symptoms.

19. Functional biliary-type pain:
    (a) Is seen after 50% of patients after cholecystectomy.
    (b) Mostly affects females.
    (c) Impaired gall bladder muscle contraction is seen.
    (d) Gall bladder ejection fraction is preserved.
    (e) Gall bladder ejection fraction less than 40% is an indication for cholecystectomy.

20. Functional dyspepsia:
    (a) Symptoms are aggravated by ingestion of the food.
    (b) Delayed gastric emptying is seen.

(c) Endoscopy is diagnostic in majority of cases.
(d) Tegaserod is useful in management.
(e) Prokinetic agents have no role in the management.

21. Functional abdominal pain syndrome:
(a) Is mostly due to malingering of symptoms.
(b) More common than inflammatory bowel syndrome.
(c) Benzodiazepines are beneficial.
(d) Cognitive behavioural therapy is beneficial.
(e) Milk-based diets are major offenders.

22. Urogenital pain:
(a) Is seen in 50% of patients.
(b) Hypertensive episodes can occur secondary to bladder distension with spinal cord injuries.
(c) Testicular pain is localised to T8–T9.
(d) Interstitial cystitis is mainly seen in the females.
(e) Levels of antiproliferative factor in urine are diagnostic of interstitial cystitis.

23. Genitourinary pain:
(a) Urethral pain syndrome has spontaneous resolution.
(b) Loin pain haematuria is a diagnosis of exclusion.
(c) Octreotide is helpful in polycystic kidney disease.
(d) History of candida is a risk factor in vulvodynia.
(e) Acupuncture is helpful in vulvodynia.

24. Obstetric pain:
(a) Pain in the first stage of labour is from the uterine body.
(b) Pain from second stage is well localised.
(c) Visceral pain in the first stage can be abolished by bilateral pudendal nerve block.
(d) Long-term oestrogen exposure increases the expression of TRPV1 afferents in the cervix.
(e) Uterine cervical distension inhibits c-fos in the spinal cord.

25. Labour pain:
(a) Can increase cardiovascular morbidities.
(b) Has no effect on respiration.
(c) Can increase gastrin and decrease gastrointestinal motility.

(d) Hypnosis is effective in 80% of patients.

(e) TENS has minimal analgesic effect.

26. Labour pain:

    (a) Entonox should be inhaled 15 s before peak uterine contraction.

    (b) Sevoflurane has better pain relief than Entonox.

    (c) Early administration of epidural in labour prolongs labour.

    (d) Neuraxial analgesia in second-stage labour increases its duration.

    (e) Programmed intermittent epidural boluses have better patient satisfaction.

27. Continuous spinal labour analgesia:

    (a) Has high incidence of neurological injuries.

    (b) High incidence of total spinal is seen.

    (c) Unintentional dural puncture is one of the indications.

    (d) Intrathecal morphine can cause hypothermia.

    (e) Has a high incidence of post-partum oral HSV reactivation.

28. Noncardiac chest pain:

    (a) Typically presents with symptoms of myocardial infarction.

    (b) Coronary artery disease is found in up to 25% of patients.

    (c) Highest prevalence is seen in females <25 years.

    (d) Proton pump inhibitors are helpful in the treatment.

    (e) Trazodone improves visceral hypersensitivity in gastroesophageal reflux disease.

29. Chronic pancreatitis:

    (a) Nerve growth factor is increased.

    (b) TRPV1 receptors are involved.

    (c) Enzyme treatment suppresses pancreatic secretion.

    (d) Lateral pancreaticojejunostomy causes complete resolution of symptoms.

    (e) Total pancreatectomy is helpful.

30. Abdominal pain wall:

    (a) Entrapment of anterior cutaneous branches is seen.

    (b) Is seen most commonly bilateral.

    (c) Increased point tenderness is seen with abdominal wall muscle contraction.

    (d) Irritable bowel syndrome is a common accompaniment.

    (e) Nerve blocks are helpful.

31. Pelvic pain:
    (a) Dyspareunia is the most common female sexual disorder.
    (b) Vulvar vestibulitis syndrome is responsive to 5% lidocaine ointment.
    (c) Dysmenorrhoea is associated with decreased levels of vasopressin.
    (d) Increased growth of endometrial cells is seen in endometriosis.
    (e) Low levels of oestrogen lead to vulvodynia.

32. Pelvic pain:
    (a) Substance P and CGRP are increased in testicular pain.
    (b) Decreased levels of tumour necrosis factor alpha in chronic prostatitis.
    (c) Pain is seen in early stage of prostatic carcinoma.
    (d) Herpes simplex virus infection can mimic pudendal neuralgia.
    (e) Coccygodynia is more common in females.

33. Pelvic pain:
    (a) Genitofemoral neuralgia presents as pain and burning sensation in inguinal region.
    (b) Dyspareunia is a feature of adenomyosis.
    (c) Pelvic venous congestion can cause pain.
    (d) Vulval pain is responsive to surgery.
    (e) Presacral neurectomy is helpful in endometriosis.

✅ Answers

1. T F F T T
   Visceral afferents mostly terminate in the spinal cord except for the vagal and glossopharyngeal ones which terminate in the brainstem. Some afferents are Aβ associated with Pacinian corpuscles in the mesentery. Convergence is a phenomenon whereby all second-order neurons that receive visceral input also receive convergent somatic input from the skin and/or muscle.

2. T T F T T
   Visceral afferents also exhibit more high affinity for nerve growth factor receptor TrKA. 70–80% of visceral dorsal root ganglion shows high reactivity for TRPV1 as against 35–60% for skin dorsal root ganglion and 40% for muscle. Visceral afferents terminate in lamina V and X. Anterior and middle insula responds to somatic stimulation.

3. F F T T F

   Most mechanosensitive afferent fibres (80%) respond at pressures less than 5 mmHg, while only 20% respond to between 20 and 30 mmHg. Silent nociceptors are seen in colon. Both serotonergic (5-HT3) and purinergic (P2X) play a role in visceral sensation.

4. F F T T F

   TRPV1 is increased in inflammatory bowel syndrome, painful bladder syndrome and vulvodynia. TRPV4 is increased along with TRPV1 in colonic hypersensitivity. Local mediators and immune competent cells are involved in functional visceral disorders.

5. F T T T T

   Visceral sensory neurons are polymodal that means they respond to multiple stimulus modalities. Gut is the main source for serotonin (95%). Visceral pain preferentially activates the perigenual portion of the anterior cingulate cortex which is an area of visceral pain and emotion.

6. T F T T T

   True visceral pain has no structural localisation, but referred visceral pain has perceived localisation to nonvisceral sites. Same segmental sites become more sensitive to inputs applied directly to those other sites. Abdominal pain is seen in 65% of females and also in the elderly. Proctalgia fugax is a sudden and severe shooting pain in rectal area that lasts for seconds/minutes and seen in 14% of patients. Levator ani syndrome is a dull ache or constant pressure that lasts for hours and seen in 7–11% of patients.

7. F T T T F

   Two sets of primary afferent fibres are seen. Bilateral anterolateral cordotomy is most useful. Sensation of visceral distension is still intact.

8. T F F T T

   Cortical stimulation is necessary for angina pain. Chemical stimuli are more effective in pericarditis. Pain after thoracotomy is mediated by phrenic nerve and blockade of the nerve gives pain relief.

9. F T F F T

   Pneumonia is associated with pleuritic pain only if peripheral parenchyma is involved. The pain when present can last up to 30 min; 25–60% of noncardiac chest pain is caused by GERD. Tietze's syndrome comprises of benign, painful and nonsuppurative localised swelling of costochondral, costoclavicular joints. Costochondritis does not present with swelling. Major cause of thoracic outlet syndrome is because of brachial plexus compression as it passes through the interscalene triangle. Venous obstruction causes outlet syndrome in 5% of patients and is due to effort-related thrombosis of axillosubclavian vein. Cyclic mastodynia is mostly seen in luteal phase and mostly present in the third decade.

10. F T T F T
Non-cyclic mastodynia is mostly unilateral and seen in the fourth decade. Post-CABG pain can present as hypoesthesia because of intercostal nerve injury, internal mammary artery dissection, placement of sternal wires presenting as hypoesthesia, hyperalgesia and allodynia. Submucosal placement of implants is twice as likely as subglandular placement to cause thoracic pain. The risk factors are female gender, young age, altered pain perception, chest wall resection and prior high levels of acute pain.

11. T F F T F
Characteristic of IBS is relief of symptoms with defaecation. The diagnostic criteria include improvement with defaecation, onset associated with change in frequency of stools and onset associated with a change in the form of stools. IBS is more common in females (2:1), and peak is seen in between 30 and 50 years. Psychiatric associations include anxiety disorder, panic disorder and PTSD. Extraintestinal manifestations include fibromyalgia, chronic fatigue syndrome, pelvic pain and dysmenorrhoea.

12. T T F T T
Infectious causes only account for 10% of the cases. Other risk factors include female sex, duration of gastroenteritis, psychological stressors, anxiety and depression.

13. T T F T T
A colorectal distending volume of approximately 60 ml evokes pain in >50% of patients (normally less than 10%). Pain in the upper gut is because of spinal nerves. Vagus nerve in upper gut causes fullness, bloating and vomiting.

14. T T F F T

Post-prandial colonic contractions cause pain in irritable bowel syndrome as against the normal. Less than normal pressures to cause pain are required as only visceral thresholds are changed and not the somatic ones. Decreased hypersensitivity to rectal stimulation is seen.

15. T T T F T

Mucosal inflammation is seen in the form of increased lamina propria cellularity with neutral infiltration. Mast cell is the main component and influences internal muscle contraction and enteric nerve excitability.

16. F F F T T

Common presentations are constipation, diarrhoea and alternating constipation and diarrhoea. Females are affected more than males (2:1). Nausea, bloating, constipation and extraintestinal symptoms are seen more in females. Risk factors include anxiety; emotional, sexual and physical abuse; stressful life events; chronic social stress; and maladaptive coping styles. Bacterial overgrowth is seen in 70–80% of patients.

17. T T T F T

Avoiding triggers like high-fat foods, raw fruits and vegetables. Patients with constipation benefit from 20 to 25 g of fibres. Alosetron (5HT3 antagonist is approved for severe IBS-D. Markers of severity include faecal incontinence, increased bowel urgency, frequent/severe pain and disability. 5HT4 agonists are useful in IBS-C, females <65. Tegaserod (5HT4 agonist) exerts its effect by stimulating peristaltic reflex and accelerating oral caecal transit. Renzapride is a combined 5HT4 agonist and 5HT3 antagonist.

18. T T F T F

Functional dyspepsia is persistent or recurrent pain or discomfort centred in the upper part of the abdomen without any organic cause. The criteria for diagnosis include bothersome post-prandial fullness, early satiation, epigastric pain, epigastric burning and no organic cause. Symptoms improve with time.

19. F T T F T

Functional biliary-type pain is seen in 20% of patients after cholecystectomy. It affects males in 80% of patients. CCK-stimulated cholescintigraphy is used to estimate gall bladder ejection fraction. The gall bladder ejection fraction is decreased in functional biliary-type pain, diabetes, pregnancy, obesity, cirrhosis and with drugs. Gall bladder ejection fraction less than 35–40% is considered to have abnormal gall bladder motility and responds well to cholecystectomy.

20. T F T T F

Delayed gastric emptying is not seen. Endoscopy has a sensitivity of 73% and a specificity of 37%. Tegaserod (5HT4 agonist and 5HT2b receptor antagonist) enhances gastric emptying. Itopride (prokinetic benzamide) has a gastrokinetic action.

21. F F T T F

Criteria for diagnosis include continuous abdominal pain, no relation to physiological events, loss of daily functioning and no evidence of malingering. Its incidence is only 2% and is seen more in females than males. There is no association of any specific diets.

22. T T F T T

Urogenital pain is seen more in females. Testicular pain is localised to T10-L1 (via superior spermatic nerve). Interstitial cystitis is seen more in females (10:1).

23. T T T F T

Urogenital pain and loin pain haematuria syndrome are seen more in females. Polycystic kidney disease is an autosomal dominant disease, and octreotide relieves pain and decreases the cyst size. The risk factors for vulvodynia are early use of oral contraceptives, early intercourse and early menarche.

24. F T F T F

Pain in the first stage is from the lower uterine segment and cervix. The second stage begins with complete cervical dilation, and pain is sharp and well localised to the vagina and perineum. The first stage of pain is relieved by bilateral paracervical plexus, while the second stage is relieved by bilateral pudendal nerve block. TRPV1 receptor antagonists reduce afferent response to cervical distension. C-fos expression is increased on cervical distension.

25. T F T F T

Labour pain can increase plasma catecholamines with an increase in cardiac output, blood pressure, peripheral vascular resistance and decreased uteroplacental blood flow. There is an associated increase in tidal volume, minute ventilation and alveolar ventilation. Labour pain can cause increase in gastric acidity and volume and delay in bladder emptying. Hypnosis is effective in only 5–10% of patients.

26. T T F T T

0.8% sevoflurane has shown better analgesic effect. Neuraxial analgesia in the second stage increases its duration by 15 min.

27. T T T T T

Continuous spinal analgesia causes more neurological injuries because of subarachnoid maldistribution of high concentration of agents. Intrathecal morphine can cause hypothermia for up to 6 h.

28. T T T T T

Highest incidence of noncardiac chest pain is seen in females between the ages of 45 and 55 years.

29. T T T F F

There is an increased release of capsaicin-evoked release of CGRP from thoracic sensory neurons. Enzyme treatment decreases pancreatic secretion and decreases intraluminal pressures thus decreasing the pain associated. Lateral pancreaticojejunostomy causes resolution in 80% of patients. Total pancreatectomy is helpful.

30. T F T T T

Entrapment of anterior cutaneous branches is seen especially of T7–T12 intercostal nerves as they pass through the rectus abdominis. It is more commonly seen on the right side. The positive Carnett test includes increased point tenderness with abdominal wall contraction.

31. T T F T T

Dyspareunia is seen in 10–15% of females. Other causes of similar pain include tampon insertion, urination and gynaecology examination. Five percent lidocaine works by blocking transmission of C fibre activity.

Increased levels of vasopressin are seen in dysmenorrhea which causes uterine ischaemia. Endometriosis is associated with increased growth of endometrial cells because of increased vascular endothelial cell growth factor. Decreased levels of oestrogen contribute to increase in number of vaginal nociceptive fibres.

32. T F F T T

Chronic prostatitis shows increased levels of TNFα along with levels of IL-1β and IL-8. Early stages of prostatic carcinoma are asymptomatic. Coccyx is more prone to trauma in females as it is less curved anteriorly and less protected by ischial tuberosities.

33. T T T F T

Genitofemoral neuralgia is exacerbated by walking, running and hyperextension of the hip. Adenomyosis is endometrial tissue in the myometrium and presents with painful and/or profuse menstruation, pain during sexual intercourse and chronic pelvic pain. Biofeedback is more helpful in vulval pain than surgery.

Cancer Pain

© Springer International Publishing AG 2018
R. Gupta, *Multiple Choice Questions in Pain Management*,
DOI 10.1007/978-3-319-56917-8_8

❓ Questions

1. Characteristics of cancer-associated pain:
   (a) Pain is often a late symptom.
   (b) Nerves are sprouting and neuroma formation may be a mechanism of action.
   (c) Mostly starts as incidental pain.
   (d) Primary afferent neurons may be sensitised directly.
   (e) Cancer cells are normally alkaline.

2. Tumour-induced bone pain:
   (a) TRPV1 antagonists can attenuate bone pain.
   (b) Cancer cells directly destroy the bone.
   (c) Osteoclast resorbs the bone by forming a highly acidic resorption bay.
   (d) Bisphosphonates decrease bone pain by decreasing osteoclast-induced acidosis.
   (e) Denosumab decreases bone pain by interfering with receptor binding of osteoclasts.

3. Mechanism of cancer pain:
   (a) Endothelins are directly nociceptive.
   (b) Endothelins play a role in tumour-induced thermal and mechanical hyperalgesia.
   (c) Tumour necrosis factor alpha antagonists have a role in heat and mechanical hyperalgesia.
   (d) IL-6 agonists decrease heat hyperalgesia.
   (e) Nerve growth factor sensitises nociceptors.

4. Molecular mechanisms of cancer pain:
   (a) Sodium channels are involved.
   (b) Anti-nerve growth factor is an intracellular event.
   (c) Macrophage infiltration of dorsal root ganglion may be seen.
   (d) Anti-nerve growth factor therapy blocks pathological sprouting of nerve fibres.
   (e) Sprouting can cause movement evoked and spontaneous breakthrough pain.

5. Mechanism of cancer pain:
   (a) Apoptosis can contribute to tumour growth.
   (b) The most common cause of pain is from nociceptors in nerves.

(c) Osseous metastases are mostly painful.
(d) Activating transcription factor-3 levels are decreased in sensory neurons of tumour cells.
(e) Osteoprotegerin decreases pain behaviour.

6. Pain associated with anticancer treatment:
   (a) Intravenous infusion causes pain because of venous spasm.
   (b) Chemical phlebitis presents as ulceration.
   (c) Cytotoxic infusion may mimic as abdominal pain.
   (d) Intraperitoneal administration of 5-fluorouracil or cisplatin is associated with pain.
   (e) Polyarthritis may be seen.

7. Pain associated with chemotherapy toxicity:
   (a) Elderly is prone to chemotherapy-induced mucositis.
   (b) Arthralgias are associated with steroid overdosage.
   (c) Taxol-induced myalgias may be reduced by steroids.
   (d) 5-Fluorouracil-induced chest pain is because of myocarditis.
   (e) Painful rash is seen with capecitabine.

8. Pain associated with hormonal treatment:
   (a) Inhibition of hormones in prostate carcinoma can cause death.
   (b) Androgen antagonist during initiation of LH-releasing hormone agonist treatment in prostate carcinoma can decrease pain.
   (c) Hormonal treatment with metastatic breast carcinoma can cause musculoskeletal pain.
   (d) High-dose vitamin D treatment can decrease aromatase inhibitor-induced arthralgia.
   (e) Interferon treatment is associated with arthralgias.

9. Pain associated with radiotherapy:
   (a) Oropharyngeal mucositis is seen with doses >4000 cGy.
   (b) Radiation enteritis is seen in 10% of patients with abdominal radiation.
   (c) Acute enteritis after abdominal radiotherapy has a good prognosis for late-onset radiation enteritis.
   (d) Pain is the most common symptom of brachial plexopathy.
   (e) Radiation myelopathy mostly involves lumbar spine.

10. Pain associated with vascular events:
    (a) Thrombosis is one of the most common causes of death in malignant disease.
    (b) Thrombotic pain associated with malignancy is seen most commonly in the feet.
    (c) Frank gangrene associated without arterial occlusion may be painless.
    (d) Superior vena cava obstruction presents with throbbing neck pain.
    (e) Pain may be seen with migratory polyarthritis.

11. Bone pain associated with malignancy:
    (a) The most common cause is infiltration of the bone cortex.
    (b) More than 50% of bone metastasis are painless.
    (c) Haematologic malignancies may present with bone pain.
    (d) Vertebral pain is most commonly seen at thoracic level.
    (e) Sacral syndrome may present as piriformis muscle syndrome.

12. Back pain associated with malignancy:
    (a) Epidural compression is mostly painless.
    (b) Epidural extension of malignancy leads to bilateral pain.
    (c) Spinal cord compression presents as central pain in a dermatomal pattern.
    (d) Spinal tenderness on percussion may be seen.
    (e) Myelography used for diagnosis may be associated with pain.

13. Characteristic of head and face pain in malignancy:
    (a) Headache is most commonly seen with anterior cranial fossa lesions.
    (b) Posterior fossa lesions often cause bifrontal headache.
    (c) Leptomeningeal metastasis is seen in >20% of systemic carcinoma.
    (d) Leptomeningeal metastasis may present as radicular buttock pain.
    (e) Middle cranial fossa involvement may present as pain in the jaw.

14. Variations of head and face pain in malignancy:
    (a) Jugular foramen syndrome may present as pain to the ipsilateral shoulder.
    (b) Vertex headache exacerbated by neck flexion is typical of occipital syndrome.
    (c) Occipital syndrome is characterised by unilateral occipital pain that worsens with neck flexion.
    (d) Sphenoid sinus metastasis may present as temporal pain.
    (e) Trigeminal neuralgia may be a manifestation of underlying neoplasm.

15. Pain associated with peripheral nervous system:
    (a) Brachial plexopathy is seen in small number of patients with plexus infiltration.
    (b) Brachial plexopathy mostly involves upper part of the plexus.
    (c) Radiation-induced brachial plexopathy presents with more intense pain.
    (d) Lumbosacral malignancy presents mostly as lower plexopathy.
    (e) Tumours in iliac crest may mimic meralgia paraesthetica.

16. Pain associated with peripheral nerve malignancy:
    (a) Upper lumbosacral plexopathy may present as a painful hip.
    (b) Radiation-induced lumbosacral plexopathy presents as radicular pain.
    (c) Paraneoplastic syndromes involve dorsal root ganglion to cause painful neuropathy.
    (d) Neoplasms mostly present with sensory neuropathies.
    (e) Idiopathic lumbosacral plexus malignancy may present as radicular pain.

17. Pain associated with visceral malignancy:
    (a) Intrahepatic metastasis may present as flank pain.
    (b) Retroperitoneal malignancy may present as upper abdominal pain.
    (c) Pancreatic cancer associated with overexpression of low-affinity receptors is associated with intense pain.
    (d) Malignant perineal pain may be associated with tenesmus.
    (e) Lung carcinoma may cause severe abdominal pain.

18. Characteristic of pain in malignancy:
    (a) Breakthrough pain is seen in <10% of patients who are on opioids.
    (b) Gynaecomastia in malignancy is associated with decreased levels of HcG.
    (c) Persistent Raynaud's phenomenon with pain is seen with germ cell tumours.
    (d) Breast cancer therapy may present as arthralgias.
    (e) Bisphosphonate therapy may present as jaw pain.

19. Pain due to complication of cancer treatment:
    (a) Is seen most intensely with chemotherapy.
    (b) Graft vs host disease may present as abdominal and limb pain.
    (c) Treatment of constipation in neutropenic patients is conservative.

(d) Granulocyte colony-stimulating factor may cause bone marrow pain.
(e) Younger children have high incidence of breakthrough pain than older children.

20. Pain assessment in children with malignancy:
    (a) Likert-based scales are most commonly used.
    (b) Pulling the ears may be a sign of pain in babies.
    (c) Observational scales have no role.
    (d) Multidimensional assessment scales are used for children between 10 and 18 years of age.
    (e) Hypertension may mimic as pain in children.

21. Effect of treatment on pain in malignancy:
    (a) Vertebral metastasis may present as neuropathic pain.
    (b) Radioisotope treatment is as effective as wide-field external beam radiotherapy in treatment of metastatic bone disease.
    (c) Chemotherapy has no role in bone pain.
    (d) Hormonal treatment is effective in metastatic bone pain because of breast carcinoma.
    (e) Bone pain relief after wide-beam external radiotherapy is over 2–4 weeks.

✔️ Answers

1. F T F T F
   Pain is mostly a common initial symptom. Seventy-five to ninty percent of patients with metastatic or advanced cancer pain will experience significant pain. Apart from nerve sprouting and neuroma formation, other mechanisms include cancer therapy, factors released from tumour, and tumour-induced nerve injury. Cancer pain starts as dull pain which gradually increases in intensity with time and then followed by incidental pain. Primary afferent neurons are sensitised by factors released by cancer cells and stromal cells. Normal cellular pH is 7.2, while cancer cells have a pH of 6.8. Osteoclasts resorb bone by generating a pH of 2–4.

2. T F T T T
   Osteoclasts produce TRPV1, and therapies that inhibit osteoclasts (bisphosphonates, denosumab) are efficacious in decreasing bone cancer pain. Cancer cells express receptor activator of nuclear factor $\kappa\beta$ ligand (RANKL) which binds to osteoclasts. Osteoclasts form an acidic bay between osteoclast and bone which can stimulate TRPV1 or ASIC3 channels and increase

bone pain. Bisphosphonates decrease osteoclast-induced acidosis thereby decreasing activation of ion-sensing TRPV1 or ASIC3 receptors that are expressed by sensory nerve fibres. Denosumab causes interference of binding of receptor activator of nuclear factor κβ ligand to receptor RANK on osteoclasts. There is complete loss of activated osteoclasts and decrease in bone pain.

3. T T T F T

Endothelin-1 may directly excite or sensitise c-fibre nociceptors. Endothelins (1, 2 and 3) are a family of vasoactive peptides that are expressed at high levels by tumours. TNFα is produced by inflammatory cells, and antagonists (etanercept) help in decreasing hyperalgesia. IL-6 action is mediated by binding to receptor IL-6R which triggers an action with transducer glycoprotein gp130. Nociceptor-specific deletion of gp130 causes decrease in heat hyperalgesia. Nociceptors activate tyrosine receptor kinase that sensitises nociceptors.

4. T F T T T

Nerve growth factor modulates the insertion of Na.v.1.8 in sensory neurons. Anti-nerve growth factor antibodies sequester extracellular nerve growth factor. Changes in dorsal ganglion include hypertrophy of satellite cells surrounding sensory neuron cell bodies, upregulation of activating transcription factor-3 and macrophage infiltration. Anti-nerve growth factor blocks pathological sprouting of sensory and sympathetic nerve fibres, and thus subsequent neuroma formation is prevented.

5. T F F F T

Apoptosis causes acidosis, and VR1 receptors are sensitised, and increase in growth of tumour is seen. The most common cause of pain is from nociceptors of soft tissues (45%), bone (35%), nerves (34%) and viscera (33%). Twenty-one percent of breast and 22% of prostate metastasis are asymptomatic. Activating transcription factor-3 is minimal in nucleus of sensory nerves which is increased in tumour cells. Osteoprotegerin is a secreted soluble receptor that is a member of the tumour necrosis factor family.

6. T F T F T

Other reasons for pain during intravenous infusion include chemical phlebitis, vesicant extravasation and anthracycline-associated flare. Chemical phlebitis (pain and linear erythema) should be distinguished from vesicant cytotoxic extravasation which presents as desquamation and ulceration. Hepatic artery infusions for hepatic metastasis may present as abdominal pain. Pain on intraperitoneal administration of 5-FU or cisplatin means suboptimal drug distribution within the abdominal cavity. Intravesical BCG treatment may cause polyarthralgia.

7. F F T F T

Younger patients are more prone to chemotherapy-induced mucositis because of higher epithelial mitotic rate. Withdrawal of steroids may result in diffuse myalgias, arthralgias and tenderness of muscles and joints. 5-Fluoruracil induces chest pain because of coronary vasospasm.

8. T T T T T

Initiation of LH-releasing hormone for prostate carcinoma can cause exacerbation of pain, spinal cord compression and sudden death. Interferon treatment is associated with fever, chills, arthralgias and headache.

9. F F F F F

Oropharyngeal mucositis is definitely seen with doses >1000 cGy, and ulceration is seen with >4000 cGy. Radiation enteritis is seen in 50% of patients and small intestine is mostly involved. Acute enteritis after radiation therapy has bad prognosis for late-onset radiation enteritis. The most common symptom after brachial plexopathy is paraesthesias along with pain and weakness. Radiation myelopathy involves mostly cervical region.

10. T F F F T

Thrombotic pain is most commonly seen in the calf but is also seen in the thigh, groin and pelvis. Phlegmasia cerulea dolens presents as ischaemia, and frank gangrene may develop without arterial or capillary occlusion and is characterised by severe pain. The superior vena cava presents as facial swelling and dilated neck veins, and pain is seen in the chest and head. Trousseau's syndrome presents with pain with migratory polyarthritis.

11. F F T F T

Bone pain is mostly associated with bone metastasis. More than 25% of bone metastasis are painless. Haematologic malignancies may present with bone pain because of replacement of the bone marrow. The most common involvement of vertebral pain is at multilevel (85%), followed by lumbosacral (20%) and cervical region (10%).

12. F F F T T

Epidural compression is symptomatic mostly and is diagnostic only in 10% of patients. Epidural extension of malignancy is mostly unilateral in the cervical and lumbosacral region, while it is bilateral in the thorax. Spinal cord compression presents as pain below the site of compression and is poorly localised with non-dermatomal dysesthesias.

13. F T F T T

Headache is most commonly seen with posterior fossa metastasis. Posterior fossa lesions cause bifrontal headache which is mostly throbbing. Leptomeningeal metastasis is seen in 1–8% of patients, most commonly seen with non-Hodgkin's lymphoma, acute lymphocytic leukaemia, adenocarcinoma of the breast and small-cell lung carcinoma. Middle cranial fossa involvement presents as pain in the jaw with signs of weakness in ipsilateral muscles of mastication.

14. T F T T T

Clivus syndrome refers to vertex headache exacerbated by neck flexion. Sphenoid sinus metastasis may present as temporal pain along with bifrontal or retroorbital pain. Trigeminal neuralgia may be a manifestation of middle or posterior cranial fossa tumours and leptomeningeal metastasis.

15. F F F T T

Brachial plexopathy is seen in more than 85% of patients especially lymphoma, lung cancer and breast carcinoma. Brachial plexopathy mostly involves the lower part (C7, 8 T1). Radiation-induced brachial plexopathy presents with less severe pain which is less common (18%). Lumbosacral malignancy presents as lower plexopathy in more than 50% of patients.

16. T F T F T

Malignant psoas syndrome may present as upper lumbosacral plexopathy, painful flexion of the ipsilateral hip and positive psoas muscle stretch test. Radiation-induced plexopathy is mostly painless. Neoplasms present with sensorimotor neuropathy and are seen mostly with Hodgkin's disease and paraproteinemias.

17. T T F T T

Pain-sensitive structures in the liver include the liver capsule, blood vessels and biliary tract. Intrahepatic metastasis presents as cholestasis causing subcostal pain or flank pain. The most common cause of retroperitoneal malignancy causing upper abdominal pain is pancreatic cancer. Pancreatic cancer associated with intense pain is associated with high-affinity receptor TrKA. Lung carcinoma may cause large adrenal metastasis causing haemorrhage and severe pain.

18. F F T T T

Breakthrough pain is seen in up to 65% of patients on opioids. Gynaecomastia is associated with increased levels of HcG. Aromatase inhibitor treatment presents as musculoskeletal pain and stiffness. Bisphosphonate treatment presents as osteonecrosis of the jaw which includes local pain, soft tissue swelling and loose teeth.

19. F T F T T

Hepatic pain in graft vs host disease is due to hepatic and intestinal inflammation and veno-occlusion. Treatment of constipation in neutropenic patients should be early and aggressive with oral laxatives. This is to prevent abdominal distension and emesis.

20. T T F T T

Likert-based scales are used with anchor points of one (no pain) and five (extreme pain). Pain in babies may manifest as pulling of ears, banging of head, flexion of knees, rigidity and clenching of fists. Gauvain-Piquard rating scale is an observational scale which is validated though with low kappa coefficients.

21. T T F F T

Chemotherapy has a defined role in bone pain especially in myeloma and breast carcinoma. Hormonal treatment has more value in metastatic bone disease pain in prostate carcinoma than in breast carcinoma.

Head and Neck Pain

© Springer International Publishing AG 2018
R. Gupta, *Multiple Choice Questions in Pain Management*,
DOI 10.1007/978-3-319-56917-8_9

❓ Questions

1. Characteristics of dental pain:
   (a) Chronic widespread pain is a risk factor.
   (b) Facial pain is derived only from teeth pulp.
   (c) Estradiol and prolactin are involved in pain sensitisation.
   (d) Dental pulp is innervated by large myelinated fibres.
   (e) Myelinated afferents innervate the whole of the teeth.

2. Characteristics of dental pain:
   (a) Inflammation of dental pulp presents as sharp stabbing pain.
   (b) Human dental pulp expresses calcitonin gene-related peptide (CGRP).
   (c) μ opioid agonists are not effective in dental pulp pain.
   (d) Pulp inflammation is prevented by good immune response.
   (e) Altered sodium channel expression is seen.

3. Characteristics of oral cancer pain:
   (a) The most common cause of malignancy is squamous cell carcinoma.
   (b) Pain is the presenting symptom.
   (c) True spontaneous pain is seen.
   (d) Oral pain may be a manifestation of treatment of breast and colon carcinoma.
   (e) Osteoradionecrosis is seen only with radiotherapy.

4. Characteristics of temporomandibular joint pain:
   (a) Generalised arthritis is one of the risk factors.
   (b) Difficulty in chewing is one of the risk factors.
   (c) Seen more in men than women.
   (d) Can be a manifestation of skeletal muscle disorder.
   (e) The most common treatment is conservative.

5. Characteristics of burning mouth syndrome:
   (a) Presents as burning pain in the lips.
   (b) May be seen secondary to diabetes.
   (c) Intermittent spasms of severe pain are seen.
   (d) Is mostly a sensory neuropathy.
   (e) Cognitive behavioural therapy is useful.

6. Characteristics of burning mouth syndrome include:
   (a) Oral mucosa shows normal appearance.
   (b) Symptoms are present for at least 2 months.

(c) Acidic foods reproduce symptoms.
(d) Dysgeusia presents as diminished ability to detect bitter flavours.
(e) Increased levels of IL-2 and IL-6 are seen.

7. Temporomandibular joint pain:
   (a) Presents as joint pain that gets relieved with rest.
   (b) Morning stiffness of jaw lasts for more than 2 h every day.
   (c) Radiologic features are not seen.
   (d) Hyaluronic injections are helpful.
   (e) Joint lavage helps relieve neuropathic pain.

8. Neurovascular headache:
   (a) Is related to the dura mater and its associated vasculature.
   (b) Vasodilation induced as a result of pain is mostly limited to ophthalmic division of trigeminal nerve.
   (c) Trigeminovascular system is involved.
   (d) Parasympathetic autonomic involvement leads to lacrimation and nasal stuffiness.
   (e) Cranial pain can cause vasodilation.

9. Characteristics of migraine:
   (a) Represents sensitivity to normal sensory input.
   (b) Familial hemiplegic migraine is because of involvement of potassium channel.
   (c) Sporadic hemiplegic migraine involves glutamate receptors.
   (d) Changes in cerebellum are seen.
   (e) SUNCT is associated with injection and tearing.

10. Diagnosis of migraine:
    (a) Is generally a continuous pain.
    (b) Aura is present in 80% of patients.
    (c) Aura is present more frequently in tension-type headache.
    (d) Migraine is seen more frequently in females.
    (e) Headache in response to triggers is characteristic.

11. Chronic daily headache:
    (a) Presents as headache for more than 6 months.
    (b) Incidence is 20%.
    (c) Headache in those >50 years old can be because of temporal arteritis.

(d) Headache worsening on supine position with Valsalva manoeuvre can occur with anterior fossa abnormalities.

(e) Medication overuse headache is one of the common reasons for daily headache.

12. Characteristics of chronic migraine headache:
    (a) Headache must respond to triptans for at least 8 days for its diagnosis.
    (b) Is seen in 20% of population.
    (c) Psychosocial factors are an association.
    (d) History of the head and neck is a major risk factor.
    (e) Typically ipsilateral autonomic features are seen.

13. Characteristics of chronic tension-type headache:
    (a) Association with depression is seen.
    (b) Is usually unilateral.
    (c) Is associated with nausea and vomiting.
    (d) Lifestyle management is the main treatment.
    (e) Topiramate is effective in treatment.

14. All are true about hemicrania continua except:
    (a) Presents as continuous headache.
    (b) Is seen more commonly in males than females.
    (c) Is usually associated with autonomic features.
    (d) Usually responds to conservative management.
    (e) Indomethacin dosage should be slowly tapered.

15. Episodic migraine:
    (a) Is seen more in males than females.
    (b) Is mostly unilateral.
    (c) Is frequently associated with vomiting.
    (d) Auras are present in 60% of patients.
    (e) Aura consists of positive features.

16. Classic migraine:
    (a) Presents with only visual auras.
    (b) Food items may precipitate migraine.
    (c) Seizures may be seen.
    (d) Triptans are effective in 100% of the population.
    (e) Symptoms become less with age.

17. Cluster headache:
    (a) Is a bilateral continuous pain.
    (b) May continue for 1 year.
    (c) High altitude may be a trigger factor.
    (d) Is not associated with autonomic features.
    (e) The diagnosis is critical.

18. Characteristics of cluster headache:
    (a) Mostly seen in females.
    (b) Autonomic features last only for the duration of the attacks.
    (c) Management is mostly conservative.
    (d) Can occur in association with trigeminal neuralgia.
    (e) Attacks can be terminated with greater occipital nerve blocks.

19. Cluster headache:
    (a) Circadian pattern is seen.
    (b) Mostly involves the maxillary area.
    (c) Aura may be present.
    (d) Females show bimodal pattern.
    (e) Surgical treatment may be required.

20. SUNCT syndrome:
    (a) Mostly unilateral headache is seen in association with cranial autonomic features.
    (b) Conjunctival tearing and injection are always seen.
    (c) Frequency of attacks can exceed up to 100/day.
    (d) Is similar to trigeminal neuralgia.
    (e) Responds to anticonvulsants.

21. Tension headache:
    (a) Is mostly bilateral.
    (b) Is seen more in females than males.
    (c) Diagnosis is based on tenderness on manual palpation.
    (d) Tricyclic antidepressants are first-line treatment for prophylaxis.
    (e) Is divided into infrequent and frequent types.

22. Pathophysiology of tension headache includes:
    (a) Increased hardness of pericranial muscles may be seen.
    (b) Tender muscles may represent central sensitisation.

   (c) Temporal or spatial summation of peripheral stimuli plays a role in headache.
   (d) Amitriptyline decreases exteroceptive silent period 2 in tension headache.
   (e) Is associated with nitric oxide supersensitivity.

23. Management of tension headache:
   (a) Tricyclic antidepressants are effective as prophylactic agents.
   (b) Botulinum toxin is helpful for chronic headaches.
   (c) Behavioural therapies have no role in the treatment.
   (d) Acupuncture has significant effect in management.
   (e) Oromandibular splints may be of help.

24. Glossopharyngeal neuralgia:
   (a) Continuous pain in the sensory division of the ninth cranial nerve is seen.
   (b) Is seen more frequently than trigeminal neuralgia.
   (c) Pain is typically seen in the distribution of glossopharyngeal nerve.
   (d) Bradycardia and cardiac arrest may be seen.
   (e) Tumours of the head and neck may cause it.

25. Treatment of glossopharyngeal neuralgia:
   (a) Anticonvulsants are the first-line treatment.
   (b) Gabapentin treatment may cause rash.
   (c) Baclofen may cause hepatic side effects.
   (d) Single glossopharyngeal nerve block usually abolishes the pain.
   (e) Management of intractable lesion is conservative.

26. Giant cell arteritis:
   (a) Pathophysiology involves vasculitis of small arteries.
   (b) Inflammatory markers are seen in 100% of patients.
   (c) May be associated with polymyalgia rheumatica.
   (d) Temporal artery biopsy shows infiltration with mononucleated cells.
   (e) Peripheral pulses may be absent.

27. Clinical features of giant cell arteritis include:
   (a) Pain is present in 100% of patients.
   (b) Prominent pulsations in the arteries are characteristic.
   (c) Visual loss is gradual.
   (d) May be accompanied with aortic dissection and rupture.
   (e) Hemiparesis may be seen.

28. Giant cell arteritis:
    (a) Giant cells on histologic examination are essential for diagnosis.
    (b) Therapy should be delayed until a diagnosis by biopsy is made.
    (c) Increased alkaline phosphatase levels may be seen.
    (d) Activated CD4 cells and macrophages contribute to the pathology.
    (e) "halo sign" is diagnostic on ultrasound.

29. Occipital neuralgias:
    (a) Mostly seen with position causing hyperextension of the head.
    (b) Continuous dull ache is typical.
    (c) Nerve blockade is diagnostic.
    (d) Radio frequency lesioning can increase the duration of pain relief.
    (e) Arnold-Chiari malformation may mimic occipital neuralgia.

30. Ocular innervation:
    (a) Sensory areas run with first division of trigeminal ganglion.
    (b) Short ciliary nerves carry postganglionic sympathetic axons.
    (c) Upper eyelid is supplied by ophthalmic nerve.
    (d) Conjunctiva is supplied by maxillary nerve.
    (e) The retina receives direct trigeminal innervation.

31. Ocular sensory innervation:
    (a) Major sensory nerves are thinly myelinated or unmyelinated.
    (b) Corneal innervation has varicosities.
    (c) Axons that penetrate corneal stroma are typically myelinated.
    (d) The number of corneal nerve terminals decreases gradually with age.
    (e) The choroid and iris are innervated by sensory nerve fibres.

32. Physiology of ocular sensory innervation:
    (a) Seventeen percent of corneal sensory nerve fibres are polymodal receptors.
    (b) Polymodal fibres fire when the temperature is more than 45°.
    (c) Fifty percent of axons innervating the cornea respond to mechanical force.
    (d) Mechanically insensitive fibres are present in the cornea.
    (e) Polymodal nociceptor and mechanonociceptor have small receptor fields.

33. Pain due to ocular disease:
    (a) Subconjunctival haemorrhage may induce severe pain.
    (b) After corneal injury, sub-basal nerve density heals faster than the epithelium.

    (c) Disturbances in cold receptor activity can contribute to pain of dry eye.

    (d) Retinitis and endophthalmitis are painful because of highly sensitive retina.

    (e) Orbital tumours are painful.

34. Ocular pain:
    (a) Retrobulbar neuritis is seen in multiple sclerosis.
    (b) Painless diplopia may be seen with cavernous sinus involvement.
    (c) Phantom eye pain is seen in significant number of patients.
    (d) Ocular pain may be associated with disappearance of corneal reflex.
    (e) Involvement of anterior segment of the eye can aggravate migraine.

✅ Answers

1. T F T T F

    Risk factors for dental pain include chronic widespread pain, age, sex (f > m) and psychosocial factors. Orofacial pain may originate from the pulp, meninges, cornea, oral and nasal mucosa and temporomandibular joint. Estradiol selectively alters gene transcription in trigeminal neurons with increased expression of neuropeptides, such as prolactin. This estradiol-dependent trigeminal system is the reason for patient sex as a risk factor. Myelinated afferents typically innervate dentine tubules, whereas unmyelinated afferents terminate in the perivascular or stromal regions of dental pulp.

2. F T F F T

    Dental hypersensitivity is due to exposed dentine tubules innervated by myelinated nociceptors causing sharp stabbing pain. Inflammation of dental pulp involves unmyelinated nociceptors causing dull ache. Human dental pulp expresses CGRP along with TRPV1.

3. T T F T F

    Pain is present in 50% of patients at the diagnosis of oral cancer and 80% at the time of diagnosis. Mostly it is associated with functional pain (chewing, talking and swallowing). Vincristine used for breast carcinoma and oxaliplatin used for metastatic colorectal carcinoma may be associated with oral pain. Osteoradionecrosis is exposed necrotic bone in the maxilla/mandible without healing >6 weeks. It is seen with intravenous bisphosphonates.

4. T T F T T

    Risk factors for temporomandibular arthritis include trauma, myofascial pain and genetic influences. Two types of temporomandibular joint dysfunction are seen: masticatory muscle disorders (majority) and articular disorders. General symptoms include difficulty in chewing, pain, earache, headache and facial pain. TMJ pain is seen more in females than males and peak is seen after 45 years of age. The pain can present as local myalgia, myofascial pain and myospasm.

5. T T F T T

    The pain and dysesthesias are mostly seen in the tongue (anterior two-thirds and tip) and intraoral soft tissues. The buccal mucosa and floor of the mouth are never involved. The systemic afflictions include diabetes, xerostomia, candidiasis and vitamin deficiency. The pain is mostly a continuous pain. It is primarily a sensory neuropathy with 60% reduction in epidermal nerve fibre density. The neuropathy is associated with positive symptoms (burning pain, dysesthesias and dysgeusia) and negative symptoms like loss of taste and paraesthesias. CBT is helpful as patients exhibit anxiety, depression and personality disorders.

6. T F T T T

    Diagnostic criteria for burning mouth syndrome include: (1) pain is persistent, (2) oral mucosa is normal and (3) no local or systemic disease. Symptoms are present for at least 4–6 months before a diagnosis can be made. Acidic foods like tomatoes and orange juice reproduce symptoms. Metallic dysgeusia is also seen (tetracycline, lithium, captopril).

7. T F F T F

    Morning stiffness usually lasts for less than 30 min along with decreased range of motion, bony enlargement and effusion. Radiologic features of osteoarthritis are seen: decreased joint space, subchondral sclerosis and subchondral cysts. Joint lavage is mostly done to increase mobility.

8. T T T T T

    The trigeminovascular system comprises of large intracranial vessels, dura mater, trigeminal nerve and second-order neurons of the trigeminal nucleus.

9. T F T F T

    Dysfunction in aminergic brainstem system leads to insensitivity to light, sound and head movement. Familial hemiplegic migraine is associated with mutation in the gene for Cav2.1 subunit of neuronal P-/Q-type voltage-gated calcium channels. Sporadic hemiplegic migraine involves glial glutamate transporter gene SLC1A3. Migraine shows changes in brainstem regions such as the dorsal midbrain and dorsolateral pons. SUNCT is short-lasting unilateral neuralgiform headache attacks with conjunctival injection and tearing.

10. F F F T T

    Migraine is mostly an episodic headache and aura is present in only 20% of patients. Aura comprises of flashing lights, zigzag lines and neurological features. Aura is not seen in tension-type headache.

11. F F T F T

    Chronic daily headache is diagnosed when there are more than 15 episodes present per month for consecutive 3 months. Incidence is 3–5%. Headache in those who are more than 50 years of age can be because of temporal arteritis, brain tumour or subdural haematoma. Headache increased with Valsalva manoeuvre is mostly due to posterior fossa tumours.

12. T F T T F

    Chronic migraine or headache is seen in 4% of patients. It is associated with depression, anxiety, fatigue, myofascial pain and gastrointestinal disorders. Risk factors include history of head and neck injury, female sex, low socioeconomic status, younger age, increased caffeine intake, obesity and stress. Autonomic features are seen in hemicrania continua presenting as redding of eye, tearing from eye, nasal congestion and rhinorrhea.

13. T F F T T

    Chronic tension-type headache is mostly bilateral and is mostly frontotemporal and/or occipitonuchal. Nausea and vomiting are not seen.

14. T F T F T

    Hemicrania continua is a continuous unilateral headache with periodic exacerbations. It is seen more commonly in females (2:1) with a mean age of 28 years. It is associated with autonomic features like tearing, conjunctival injection, nasal congestion, ptosis, eyelid oedema and miosis. Most common areas involved are occipital and frontal areas. The pain usually responds to indomethacin as prophylactic agent.

15. F T F F T

    Episodic migraine is seen more in females (18%) than males (6%) and mostly between the ages of 20–45 years. It is mostly unilateral and lasts between 4 and 72 h. Vomiting is a feature of childhood or adolescent migraine. Auras are present in about 20% of patients and last between 5 and 60 min. The most common aura seen is visual followed by sensory auras. Auras are mostly positive features like flickering lights, spots and scotomas, while small number of patients present with negative features like blurriness or loss of vision in a hemifield.

16. F T T F T

    Visual auras are predominantly seen. Other auras seen include sensory (pins and needles, numbness), speech (dysphasia) and motor (hemiplegia). The triggers for migraine include changes in sleep pattern, skipping meals, stress, change in weather and foods (red wine, cheese) and caffeine. Triptans are effective in two-thirds of population. Symptoms become less as males approach 50 and females approach menopause.

17. F T T F T

    Cluster headache is mostly unilateral which lasts for 1 h and may occur up to eight times a day. Nocturnal attacks are typical. Twenty percent of patients experience chronic episodes for up to 1 year without remission periods of 4 weeks or longer. Trigger factors include high altitude, tobacco use, alcohol and obstructive sleep apnoea. It is usually associated with autonomic features like lacrimation, rhinorrhoea, conjunctival injection, ptosis, miosis and periorbital oedema. Diagnosis is mostly clinical while atypical cases are diagnosed with MRI.

18. T F F T T

    Cluster headache is mostly seen in females than males (7:3). It is mostly seen in the third to fourth decade. Autonomic features may persist and can last after the attack especially Horner's syndrome. Partial Horner's syndrome may be seen which includes miosis and ptosis without anhidrosis. Subcutaneous sumatriptan is the drug of choice and is contraindicated in ischaemic heart disease. Other effective therapies include oxygen and lidocaine 10%. Prevention for cluster attacks is achieved by verapamil, lithium, methysergide, steroids and melatonin. Cluster-tic syndrome is when cluster headache is associated with trigeminal neuralgia.

19. T F T T T
Cluster headache is seen between midnight and 02:00 am. The headaches are maximally seen between the months of February and June. Cluster headache mostly involves ophthalmic division (90%). The symptoms are also seen in maxillary and mandibular distribution (lower-half syndrome). Mostly visual auras may be seen. Females show bimodal pattern at the ages of 20 years and 50 years. Effective therapy includes trigeminal nerve resection which involves interruption of autonomic patterns.

20. T F T F T
SUNCT is short-lasting unilateral neuralgiform headache attacks with conjunctival injection and tearing. SUNA is the same syndrome in the absence of conjunctival injection and tearing. Up to 200 attacks may be seen per day which involve strictly unilateral, severe, neuralgiform attacks in ophthalmic division of the trigeminal nerve. The attacks usually last for 5–120 s. SUNCT attacks are mostly in distribution of the ophthalmic nerve, while trigeminal neuralgia involves ophthalmic division in less than 5% of patients. SUNCT attacks are longer, have autonomic symptoms and have a refractory period. SUNCT usually responds to lamotrigine and topiramate.

21. T T T T T
Tension headache is mostly bilateral, pressing, non-pulsating and mild to moderate with no aggravation on physical exercise and no aura. Diagnosis is based on tenderness on palpation over seven locations (frontal, temporal, masseter, pterygoid, sternocleidomastoid, splenius and trapezius muscles) with pain scores between 0 and 3. Infrequent type presents with episodes occurring less than 1/month.

22. T T T T T
Qualitatively altered nociception from tender muscles most likely reflects central sensitisation of second-order nociceptors in patients with chronic myofascial pain. Painful stimuli in trigeminal territory induce two successive suppressions of voluntary EMG activity in jaw muscles (ES1 and ES2) mediated by interneurons. Inhibitory interneurons mediating ES2 are inhibited by serotonergic pathways and activated by nicotinic cholinergic

mechanism. Nitric oxide administration causes decrease in headache and muscle tenderness.

23. T T F F T

Botulinum toxin A is helpful in the treatment. Behavioural therapies such as relaxation and biofeedback have definite role.

24. F F F T T

Continuous pain is not seen but paroxysms of pain are seen. Glossopharyngeal neuralgia resembles trigeminal neuralgia but is 100 times less frequent. Pain may also be seen in vagus and trigeminal areas in 20% of patients (overflow pain). Overflow of these neural impulses to the vagus nerve may cause bradycardia, syncope and cardiac arrest. Tumours of cerebellopontine angle may cause pain which is dull aching persisting between paroxysms of tic-like pain.

25. T T T F F

Carbamazepine is the first-line treatment and shows rapid response. Gabapentin treatment causes rash, dizziness, sedation and confusion. Sequential glossopharyngeal nerve blocks are required for the treatment. Management is mostly surgical (Janetta technique) which involves micro-vascular decompression of the glossopharyngeal root.

26. F F T F T

Giant cell arteritis involves medium and large arteries (near the arch of the aorta) that affects patients more than 50 years old. It is seen more in females than males (3:1). Two to ten percent of patients have normal ESR. Temporal arteritis biopsy may show vasculitis characterised by predominance of mononuclear cell infiltration or granulomatous inflam-mation associated with multinucleated giant cells. Ten to fifteen percent of patients have negative biopsies. Aortic arch syndrome presents as decreased or absent peripheral pulses, discrepancies in blood pressure and the presence of arterial bruits.

27. F F F T T

Headache is predominantly temporal and seen in two-thirds of patients. Vessels are thickened, tender and nodular with absent or decreased pulsations. Giant cell arteritis may present with sudden, painless and per-manent blindness. Cilioretinal artery may be occluded causing anterior ischaemic neuropathy. It may be associated with aortic dissection and rupture in 10–15% of patients. Neurological manifestations include hemiparesis, peripheral neuropathy, deafness, depression and confusion, and non-neurological manifestations include myocardial infarction, aortic regurgitation and congestive cardiac failure.

28. F F T T T
Giant cells (small cells with 2–3 nuclei up to masses of 100 mm containing many nuclei) are not seen in all sections and are not diagnostic. Biopsy should be done before steroid treatment as inflammatory cell infiltrate may be reduced, but treatment should be started before histologic diagnosis. Liver biopsy shows portal and intralobar inflammation with focal liver cell necrosis and small epithelial cell granuloma. Activated CD4 and macrophages disrupt internal elastic lamina by releasing metalloproteinases. In adventitia, IL-1 and IL-6 are released. Inflamed temporal arteritis shows a concentric hypoechogenic mural thickening (halo) representing inflammatory wall oedema.

29. T F T T T
Occipital neuralgias present as persistent pain at the base of the skull with sudden shock like paraesthesia in distribution of greater and lesser occipital nerves. The diagnosis is by nerve blockade.

30. T T T T F
Sensory axons move with ophthalmic nerves, enter the superior orbital fissure and branch into nasociliary, frontal and lacrimal nerves. Long ciliary nerves comprise mainly of main sensory output of the globe. The upper eyelid is supplied by the frontal nerve.

31. T T F T T
Nerves supplying the cornea terminate as free nerve endings that have enlargements along their myelin sheath. Normally corneal nerve terminals are about 600/sqmm which decrease with age.

32. F F F T F
Seventy percent of corneal sensory fibres are polymodal nociceptors. Most of them are C fibres. Polymodal fibres fire when the temperature is between 30° and 40° but also when the temperature is less than 29°. Fifteen to twenty percent of peripheral axons innervating the cornea respond only to mechanical stimuli and are responsible for acute, sharp sensation of pain. There are mechanical insensitive fibres in the cornea

called silent fibres which are unresponsive to cooling. Polymodal noci-ceptor and mechanonociceptor fibres have large receptor fields. Cold receptors have small fields.

33. F F T F F

Subconjunctival haemorrhage causes mild pain, whereas inflammation of episclera and sclera may cause intense pain. Epithelium heals rapidly within a few days, whereas sub-basal nerve density recovers up to 65% in 3–4 weeks. Sensory inflow from cold thermoreceptors of the ocular surface helps maintain basal tear flow. The retina is not sensitive, and pain is mostly seen only on simultaneous involvement of the uveal tract. Orbital tumours are painless unless they become infiltrated by blood vessels or cause orbital haemorrhage.

34. T F T T T

Optic neuritis is seen along with retrobulbar neuritis in multiple sclerosis. Inflammatory conditions of the cavernous sinus near the superior orbital fissure present as pain, diplopia and paralysis of extraocular muscles (Tolosa-Hunt syndrome). Phantom eye pain is seen in about 26% after nucleation. Disappearance of corneal reflex is seen in Horton's neuralgia. This includes trigeminal neuralgia and hyperemia. It has hereditary tendency and gender dependence.

Miscellaneous

© Springer International Publishing AG 2018
R. Gupta, *Multiple Choice Questions in Pain Management*,
DOI 10.1007/978-3-319-56917-8_10

❓ Questions

1. Chronic pain in paediatrics:
    (a) Persistent pain is seen in 10% of patients.
    (b) Children's anxiety sensitivity index is a better predictor of pain.
    (c) Pain-related functional disability is seen more in boys.
    (d) Relaxation and cognitive behavioural therapy has no role in paediatric chronic pain.
    (e) Parental attention decreases the symptoms in paediatric chronic pain.

2. Complex regional pain syndrome in paediatrics:
    (a) Allodynia, hyperalgesia and loss of function are seen.
    (b) Upper extremity is commonly involved.
    (c) The incidence is equal in males and females.
    (d) Cognitive behavioural therapy has no role.
    (e) Peripheral small nerve fibre neuropathy has been implicated.

3. Neuropathic pain in paediatrics:
    (a) CRPS 1 can occur in both the extremities at the same time.
    (b) Tactile allodynia in the absence of skin problems is characteristic.
    (c) Hyperalgesia seen is typically to warmth.
    (d) Quantitative sensory testing has no role in diagnosis of CRPS.
    (e) Decrease in bone scan isotope uptake is seen.

4. Headache in paediatrics:
    (a) Headache seen in childhood progresses to a headache-free state in adulthood.
    (b) Chronic daily headache lasts for > than 8 h daily.
    (c) Sleep deprivation is common.
    (d) The most common is tension-type headache.
    (e) Neuropathic headache is occasionally present.

5. Chest pain in children:
    (a) Mostly seen in females.
    (b) The most common cause is chest wall pain.
    (c) The most common cause of chest wall pain is osteochondritis.
    (d) The most common cardiac cause is mitral valve prolapse.
    (e) Gastroesophageal reflux disease is rarely seen.

6. Visceral pain in children:
   (a) Seen in 25% of paediatric population.
   (b) Is seen more in females.
   (c) Fibre intake increases pain.
   (d) Lactose intolerance may cause abdominal pain.
   (e) Cognitive behavioural therapy may help.

7. Chronic pain in elderly:
   (a) Seen more in males.
   (b) Decreased concentration of GABA and serotonergic receptors is seen.
   (c) Topical nonsteroidal analgesics have no advantage over oral preparations.
   (d) Opioid users are more prone to fractures.
   (e) Cognitively impaired patients may underreport pain.

8. Pain in pregnancy:
   (a) Critical period for avoiding analgesics is from conception to tenth menstrual week of pregnancy.
   (b) Nonsteroidal analgesics have no direct teratogenic effects.
   (c) Breast-feeding contributes to 10–15% of neonatal dose of medications.
   (d) Nonsteroidal analgesic use can cause narrowing of ductus arteriosus.
   (e) High-dose aspirin therapy increases the risk of intracranial haemorrhage in neonates born <35 weeks.

9. Analgesics in pregnancy:
   (a) Chronic opioid usage in pregnancy is associated with low birth weight and decreased head circumference.
   (b) Abrupt cessation of opioids in pregnancy has no effect on foetus.
   (c) Methadone is compatible with breast-feeding.
   (d) Females who are on methadone have lower incidence on neonatal abstinence syndrome.
   (e) Buprenorphine is not recommended during pregnancy.

10. Analgesics in pregnancy:
    (a) Mepivacaine can cause teratogenicity.
    (b) Steroids have no effect on breast-feeding.
    (c) Benzodiazepines are safe in first trimester.
    (d) Antidepressants are not excreted into human milk.
    (e) Anticonvulsants are safe during pregnancy.

11. Pain in pregnancy:
    (a) Caffeine intake has no effect on foetus.
    (b) Sumatriptan is safe in pregnancy and breast milk.
    (c) Transient osteoporosis of the hip may cause pain.
    (d) Low back pain seen peaks at 36th weeks.
    (e) TENS can be used during pregnancy.

12. Migraine during pregnancy:
    (a) Symptoms decrease during the pregnancy.
    (b) New onset is usually seen in the first trimester.
    (c) Antiphospholipid syndrome is a differential diagnosis.
    (d) Ergot preparations are safe during pregnancy.
    (e) Post-partum headaches are rare.

13. Adult haemoglobin:
    (a) Is a pentamer of alpha and globin chains.
    (b) Haeme moiety carries oxygen.
    (c) Haemoglobinopathies are because of haemoglobin-B.
    (d) The most common variant of sickle cell disease is HB-C.
    (e) Haemoglobinopathies are inherited in autosomal codominant manner.

14. Pain in sickle cell disease:
    (a) Polymer formation is the main mechanism.
    (b) Central sensitisation is involved because of repetitive vaso-occlusion.
    (c) Begins after 5 years of life as foetal haemoglobin is replaced.
    (d) Hand and feet pain is a characteristic.
    (e) Vaso-occlusive episodes are less frequent in childhood.

15. Vaso-occlusive episodes:
    (a) Are seen mostly in childhood.
    (b) Episodes last for up to 2–3 h.
    (c) Multiple bones are involved simultaneously.
    (d) Mental health issues may be associated.
    (e) Both recurrent and chronic pain may be seen.

16. Causes of pain in sickle cell disease:
    (a) Visceral pain is uncommon.
    (b) Cholelithiasis or bile duct obstruction pain is seen more in children.
    (c) Avascular necrosis is only seen in vertebral column.

(d) Leg ulcers are seen in adults.
(e) Triptans are the drug of choice for migraine in sickle cell disease.

17. Management of pain in sickle cell disease:
    (a) Home setting is ideal for acute pain management.
    (b) Codeine is the ideal analgesic.
    (c) Vaso-occlusive pain will require strong opioids.
    (d) Intravenous nalbuphine is ideal in sickle cell disease as it has less side effects.
    (e) Parenteral nonsteroidal analgesics should be avoided.

18. Pain management in sickle cell disease:
    (a) Demand mode of patient-controlled analgesia is more likely to give pain relief than continuous pain.
    (b) Refractory sickle cell pain is seen after 10 days.
    (c) Psychological support is useful.
    (d) Chronic daily pain requires long acting opioids.
    (e) Vaso-occlusive pain has a single target for analgesic management.

19. Acute chest syndrome in sickle cell disease:
    (a) Presents with a clear X-ray.
    (b) Level of haemoglobin is maintained.
    (c) Fat bodies may be seen in sputum or urine.
    (d) Transfusion may be required.
    (e) Pulmonary failure with cor pulmonale may be seen.

20. Acute splenic sequestration in sickle cell disease:
    (a) Fall in reticulocyte count is seen.
    (b) Spleen may be shrivelled.
    (c) Hypovolemia may be seen.
    (d) May mimic sudden infant death syndrome.
    (e) Acute sequestration is an indication for splenectomy.

21. Acute burn injury pain:
    (a) Is due to thermal tissue injury to sensory organs.
    (b) The dermis is destroyed in third-degree burns, so they are painless.
    (c) All burn injuries that involve the dermis can sensitise both mechano-receptors and dorsal root ganglion.
    (d) Pain can be predicted based on the grade of the injury.
    (e) Generalised continuous background pain is seen.

22. Management of burn pain:
    (a) Sedation has better evidence with opioids for procedural pain.
    (b) Breakthrough pain management can be because of predictable changes in the burn wound.
    (c) Management of post-operative pain may be helpful with the use of strong non-pharmacological interventions.
    (d) Nursing assessment of the burn pain is the ideal pain assessment tool.
    (e) Intramuscular administration of opioids should be avoided.

23. Anaesthesia in burns pain:
    (a) Entonox is an effective analgesic.
    (b) Risk of emergency delirium is significant in oral ketamine use.
    (c) Inhaled sevoflurane is also effective in procedural pain.
    (d) Topical agents are less useful.
    (e) Propofol is safe.

24. Pain management in burns:
    (a) Opioid requirements may be increased.
    (b) Infectious complications may be increased.
    (c) Methadone is not effective in burns patients.
    (d) Ketamine is seen to decrease wind-up.
    (e) Alpha-2 agonists have opioid-sparing effects.

25. Pain management in emergency department:
    (a) Chronic pain management is seen up to 5% of patients.
    (b) The most effective assessment scale is graphic rating scale.
    (c) Risk factor for undertreatment is extreme age.
    (d) Mixed agonist/antagonist has ceiling effect on both analgesia and respiratory depression.
    (e) Tramadol-acetaminophen combination is effective.

26. Pain in intensive care unit:
    (a) Incidence is only 10%.
    (b) Early offset of action of fentanyl makes it an ideal agent as an analgesic.
    (c) The early use of analgesics decreases rate of complications in intensive care.
    (d) Pain in critically ill and post paediatric patients is helpful.
    (e) FLACC scale is more useful for assessment of pain.

27. Pain management in intensive care:
    (a) Patients do not have fear of addiction.
    (b) Pain relief may lead to early recovery.
    (c) Epidural neuraxial anaesthesia improves most of pulmonary function tests in the post-operative period.
    (d) Opioids diminish stress response because of efferent nerve blockade of adrenal medulla.
    (e) Ketorolac has inherent advantage of being able to be used for more than 1 week.

✅ Answers

1. T F F F F
    Persistent pain is seen in 5–10% of patients. Children's anxiety sensitivity index is a better predictor of health-related quality of life. Pain-related functional disability is seen more in girls than boys. Parental attention increases the symptoms in abdominal pain.

2. T F F T T
    Lower extremity is commonly involved in CRPS. It is seen more in females than males and peak is seen between 11 and 13 years.

3. T T F F T
    Hyperalgesia seen is typically to cold. QST has a role in CRPS 1.

4. T F T T T
    Chronic headaches occur at least 15 times/month for a period of 3 months and can last for 4 h daily. Tension-type headache is mostly seen with complains of frontotemporal or frontoparietal headaches. Headaches are seen because of contraction of the temporalis muscle. Neuropathic headache is seen after ventriculo-peritoneal shunt insertion and surgical decompression for a Chiari malformation.

5. F T T T F
    Chest pain in children is seen mostly in males with a peak at 13 years. The most common cause is chest wall pain (65%), cardiac (5%), respiratory (13%) and psychological (9%). Most common abdominal cause of chest pain is GERD.

6. F F F T T
    Visceral pain is seen in 10–15% of paediatric population. It is predominantly equal both in males and females. Fibre intake decreases the pain by 50%.

7. F T F T T
    Risk factors for increased pain in elderly are female gender, increased age, low income, depression and anxiety. C and Aδ functions decreased in elderly. Topical nonsteroidal analgesics are better tolerated and have few side effects compared to the oral preparations.

8. T T F T T
    Nonsteroidal analgesics may cause delay in the onset of labour, decreased amniotic fluid and risk of newborn of pulmonary hypertension and renal injury. Breast-feeding contributes to 1–2% and early breast-feeding poses little risk. If nonsteroidal analgesics are required in pregnancy, usage should be limited to <48 h. Usage should be discontinued by 34 weeks gestation to avoid pulmonary hypertension in newborn.

9. T F T T T
    Abrupt cessation of opioids in pregnancy leads to withdrawal syndrome (foetal tachycardia and death). Neonatal abstinence syndrome is associated with irritability, increased tone, poor feeding and seizures. The incidence is 30–90%. Incidence is only 11% with pregnant females on methadone.

10. T T F F F
    Mepivacaine can cause toxicity while bupivacaine and lignocaine have no effect. Benzodiazepines increase the risk of cleft palate and congenital inguinal hernia. If administered immediately before delivery, it can increase risk of foetal hypothermia, hyperbilirubinemia and respiratory depression. Anticonvulsants if given in the first trimester are associated with neural tube effects, facial clefts, hypospadias and small for gestational age babies (carbamazepine, cleft palate; topiramate, cleft lip/palate).

11. F T T T T
    Caffeine causes decrease in foetal heart rate, increased frequency of heart rate accelerations, increased incidence of supraventricular tachycardia and atrial flutter. Transient osteoporosis of the hip causes pain, limitation of hip movement and osteoporosis of the femoral head. Low back pain starts at 18 weeks and is due to direct pressure of foetus on lumbosacral nerves on the lumbar plexus. TENS can increase the risk of inadvertent induction of labour and foetal cardiac conduction abnormalities.

12. T T T F F

Migraine improves in 50–80% of patients in pregnancy, and no improvement is seen after the second trimester. Choriocarcinoma and cocaine ingestion are differential diagnosis. Ergot increases uterine tone and placental flow causing abortion. Post-partum headaches are seen in 30–40% of patients. It is due to rapid ovarian withdrawal of progesterone and estradiol.

13. F T F F T

Adult haemoglobin is a tetramer of 2 α and 2 β globin chains ($\alpha2\beta2$). The most common variant is HB-S. There is a single base mutation in the sixth codon of exon 1 of the β globin. In HB-S, glutamic acid is replaced by valine, while in HB-C, glutamic acid is replaced by lysine.

14. F T F T F

The mechanisms of pain in sickle cell disease include polymer formation; adhesion of sickled erythrocytes, leucocytes and platelets; and abnormal vascular endothelium. Pain starts within a years time as foetal haemoglobin gets replaced. Hand and foot syndrome becomes less prevalent in older children and rare after 5–7 years. Vaso-occlusive episodes are seen with increased frequency during childhood.

15. T F F T T

Vaso-occlusive episodes are seen in childhood, adolescence and young adults. Episodes last between 2 and 3 days. A small number of body sites are involved at a time which are mostly the lower legs, back and chest.

16. F T F F F

Acute left upper quadrant visceral pain may be seen from enlargement of splenic capsule. Episodic right upper quadrant colicky pain and jaundice is seen in cholelithiasis and may need cholecystectomy. Avascular necrosis is also seen in shoulders and hips. Leg ulcers are rarely seen in paediatric population and are over the medial malleolus of either or both ankles. Triptans are not used in sickle cell disease because of the cardiovascular concerns. Typically migraine is not seen but the headache seen is a mix of migraine, tension headache and chronic daily headache.

17. T F T F T

Treatment of acute pain in home setting is ideal as it is more comforting for children and is least likely to be disruptive to the family's normal activities and routine. Codeine is not ideal as it does not have good efficacy and mostly mild analgesics are helpful.

18. F F T F F
Cognitive behavioural therapy in the form of guided imagery and calming self-talk is also helpful in addition to the pharmacologic therapy.

19. F F T T T
Acute chest syndrome may present with fever and respiratory symptoms accompanied by new pulmonary infiltrates on chest X-ray.

20. F F T T F
There is an increase in reticulocytes with a decrease in haemoglobin and platelets. There is a sudden increase in spleen size which is the characteristic. Acute sequestration responds to transfusion of sickle negative red cells, while after the acute event stabilisation, splenectomy is helpful in preventing further attacks.

21. T F T F F
There is an additional acute inflammatory response contributing to the pain. Full thickness or third-degree burns have total loss of the dermis but can still be painful, though hypalgesia to stimulation is common.

22. T T T F T
Procedural pain is significantly more intense but is of shorter duration, so the combination of sedation and morphine is ideal. Breakthrough pain management can be altered because of the predictable changes involved in the form of proliferation of epidermal skin buds during multiple interventions. Post-operative pain most commonly is because of newly created graft wound harvesting sites; therefore information provision is necessary, so that patients can anticipate both the increase and the temporary nature of post-operative pain. Intramuscular administration of opioids is unhelpful because of unpredictable vascular absorption from various compartments and inadequate muscle perfusion.

23. T T T F T
Entonox is a mix of 50% nitrous oxide and 50% oxygen, and side effects include spontaneous abortion and bone marrow suppression. The side effects are minimally seen in burn pain management. Emergency delirium is seen in 5–30% of population, especially more in the elderly. EMLA up to a maximum of 2 g is safe and can be used, while 5% lignocaine ointment at 1 mg/sq cm has offered analgesic effect.

24. T T F T T

    Higher opioid requirements are seen because of acute opioid tolerance. Methadone is helpful as it is long acting. The risk of complications is increased because of the immunosuppressant effect of opioids. Methadone is especially useful in burns patients with opioid tolerance and has neuropathic pain. Ketamine decreases the wind-up and thus reduces the area of secondary hyperalgesia. Alpha-2 agonists decrease norepinephrine release at presynaptic receptor sites causing sympatholysis and thus decreasing autonomic outflow.

25. F F T T T

    Forty percent of patients attending emergency department have some form of pain. Numerical rating scale is sensitive to the short-term changes in pain intensity associated with emergency care. Graphic rating scale is for paediatric population. Undertreatment (oligo-analgesia) is a common accompaniment in emergency department, and risk factors include extreme age and minority ethnicity.

26. F F F T F

    Pain in intensive care is seen in 60–75% of patients. Fentanyl has rapid onset of action which makes it ideal, but on prolonged infusion, lipophilicity contributes to prolonged offset of action. The use of analgesia is accompanied by increased incidence of haemodynamic instability, more mechanical ventilation and longer intensive care stay. The Face, Legs, Activity, Cry and Consolability scale is mainly used for paediatric setting. The scale validated for intensive care unit is critical care pain observation tool (CPOT).

27. F T F T F

    A fear of addiction is seen on 20% of patients in intensive care. There is no evidence of neuraxial anaesthesia on pulmonary function tests (FEV1, FVC, PEFR). Opioids diminish stress response by decreasing hyperglycaemic and adrenergic response. Ketorolac should not be used for more than 5 days because of the side effects like gastric mucosal hypoperfusion, platelet aggregation and renal perfusion.

Supplementary Information

Bibliography – 154

© Springer International Publishing AG 2018
R. Gupta, *Multiple Choice Questions in Pain Management*,
DOI 10.1007/978-3-319-56917-8

Bibliography

Benzon HT. Practical Management of pain. Mosby (2013)

Bruera ED, Portenoy RK. Cancer pain assessment and management. Cambridge University Press (2009)

Marcus DA. Headache and chronic pain syndromes. Humana press (2007)

Wall and Melzack's textbook of pain. Saunders (2013)

Pasricha PJ, Willis WD, Gebhart GF. Chronic abdominal and visceral pain:theory and practice. CRC Press (2006)

Piekartx JMV. Craniofacial pain: Neuromusculoskeletal assessment, Treatment and Management. Butterworth- Heinemann (2007)

Walsman SD. Pain Review 2nd ed. Elsevier (2016)

Printed in the United States
By Bookmasters